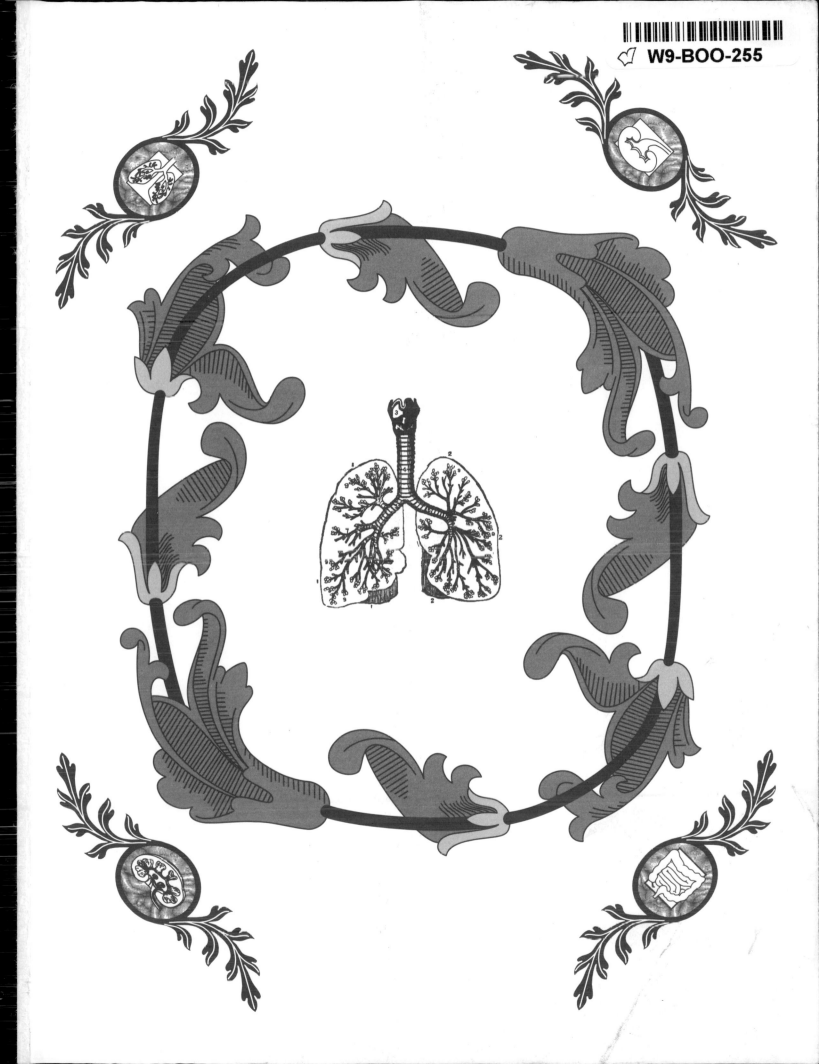

Editors: A. Juno & V. Vale
Production Manager: Kim Lenox
Book Design: A. Juno
Consultant: Ken Werner
Thanks to: C. Francesca Tussing, the Spinrad family

Editorial address for RE/Search Publications and Juno Books:
A. Juno
111 Third Avenue, #11G
New York, NY 10003
tel: 212-388-9924, fax: 212-388-1151, e-mail: ajuno@junobooks.com

For à catalog send 6 stamps to:
Juno Books / powerHouse Books
180 Varick Street, Suite 1302
New York, NY 10014-4606
www.JunoBooks.com / www.powerHouseBooks.com

US BOOKSTORE *and* NON-BOOKSTORE DISTRIBUTION:
powerHouse Cultural Entertainment, Inc.
180 Varick Street, Suite 1302
New York, NY 10014-4606
tel: 212 604 9074, fax: 212 366 5247, e-mail: orders@powerhousebooks.com

U.K. DISTRIBUTION:
Turnaround
Unit 3, Olympia Trading Estate
Coburg Road
London N22 6TZ, United Kingdom
tel: 0181 829 3000, fax: 0181 881 5088, e-mail: sales@turnaround-uk.com

ITALY DISTRIBUTION:
Logos Art srl
Via Curtatona 5/f
41100 Modena Loc. Fossalta, Italy
tel: 059 41 87 11, fax: 059 28 16 87, e-mail: logos@books.it

BENELUX DISTRIBUTION:
Nilsson & Lamm
Pampuslaan 212, Postbus 195
1380 AD Weesp, The Netherlands
tel: 02 94 494949, fax: 02 94 494455, e-mail: g.boor@nilsson-lamm.nl

Printed in Hong Kong by Colorcraft Ltd.
10 9 8 7 6 5 4 3

Permission granted to reprint quotes from the following:
Martin, Judith, *Miss Manners' Guide to Excruciatingly Correct Behavior.* New York, New York: Warner Books, Inc., 1983.
Montaigne, Michel de, *The Complete Essays of Montaigne* (tr. Donald M. Frame). Stanford, California: Stanford University Press, 1958.
Pirsig, Robert, *Zen and the Art of Motorcycle Maintenance.* New York, New York: William Morrow and Company, Inc., 1974.

Cover Illustration (front and back): Phoebe Glockner

The RE/Search
GUIDE
TO
BODILY
FLUIDS

by Paul Spinrad

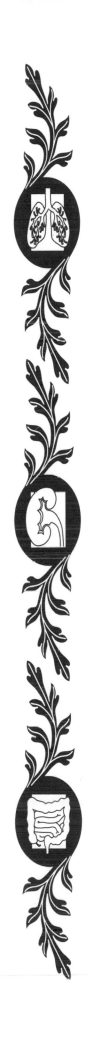

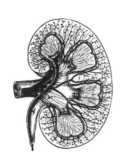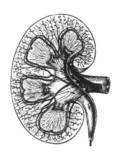

CONTENTS

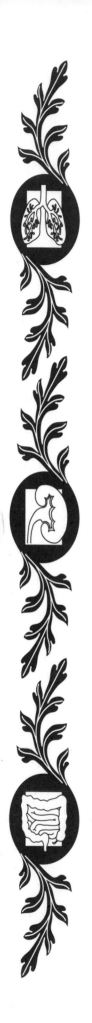

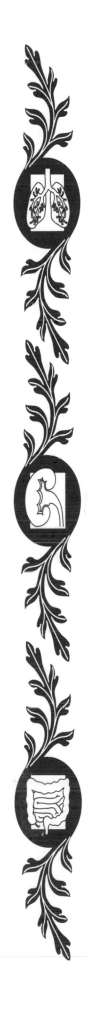

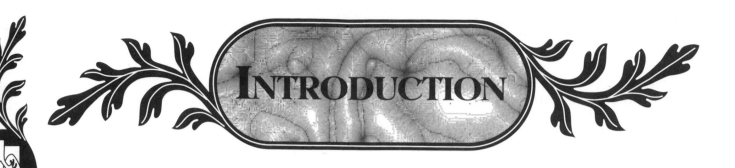

INTRODUCTION

'... a radical rethinking of our relationship with nature'

From Victorian times well into this century, American magazines carried advertisements extolling the advantages of "silent flush" toilets. The idea was that if you were playing bridge with friends at home and the urge to excrete came, you could excuse yourself with some polite lie about wanting to check on the canary, attend to the horrid task, and then return to the table without anyone knowing where you'd been. If you lacked a "silent flush" model, however, the sound of the toilet would jar the guests to the realization that the "go check on the canary" story was a lie, and that you had just wanted to take a leak or pinch a loaf after all. That hideous sound of common plumbing would brand you a liar and remind everyone of their mortality, letting you know that no matter how ready your minds and souls are to live in an eternal abstract world of language, reason, truth, beauty, and card games, you're still trapped inside aging meat machines.

Broadcast television constantly shows us murders, rapes, and dozens of other crimes which rarely, if ever, touch most of us directly. Records, books, and magazines can be even more explicit. The scatological, however, which affects all of us at all ages, is taboo. A perfectly healthy area of our lives, immediately comprehensible to anyone, can never be shown on television and is all but ignored by media which otherwise stop at nothing. Why?

Meanwhile, artists and writers who do draw upon the scatological, such as Andres Serrano and James Joyce, become centers of controversy. They're dragged into courtrooms and hearings and forced to defend their work against people shocked and offended as only people who are trying to escape from something within themselves can be. And all over things every three-year-old knows about and has no aversion to. What's going on here?

Many cultures in many times have used human excreta as components of medicines and magic potions. But it is in our culture today that these materials have the greatest magical power. We rarely mention them, but when we do, the effect can be electric. They're some of the commonest substances around, and yet because of what they represent to us and remind us of, they repel, shock, and offend. They're a part of us, literally inside of us all, but our collective reaction against them and against people who view them differently has motivated us to wage war, commit genocide, and destroy the environment. That's a lot of magic power. Magic power we could do without.

Erich Fromm, Norman O. Brown, and others, drawing on Freud, have suggested that our society denies bodily functions because collectively, we have an anal personality. Long ago, we repressed bodily desires in exchange for objectivity, industry, punctuality, and thrift. We prospered as a result, subjugating and controlling other less repressed societies and nature itself (locally, at least) with our science and technology. In exchange, however, we lost our comfort with ourselves and with life as a whole. Reminders of our past, our origins, our biology, disturb us deeply, and we, as people and as nations, constantly fight against those who threaten our fragile self-images.

At the same time, our reluctance to accept our oneness with nature has also brought us to the brink of worldwide ecological disaster. Our denial of nature grows from deep religious and cultural roots, so unfortunately, as Al Gore asserts in *Earth in the Balance* (1992), only a radical rethinking of our relationship with nature can save the earth's ecology for future generations.

I believe that radical rethinking starts at home. How can we realign with nature globally if we can't even do it with our own bodies?

In *Life Against Death* (1959), Norman O. Brown also argues that we will all risk death if we don't throw over our repression and begin once again to embrace life. Centuries of anality have given us knowledge, social structures, and technologies which we could use, if we chose to, to reengineer our place in the world and allow everyone to enjoy healthy lives on a healthy planet well into the future. Right now, however, anal traits such as greed and obstinacy discourage us from making this new choice.

Obviously, *The Re/Search Guide to Bodily Fluids* is suitable bathroom reading, and I think the bathroom is a fine place to keep it. Part of my aim in writing it, however, is to bring bodily functions out of the (water) closet and into the open, into polite conversation and if I'm successful, you won't reflexively relegate the book to the magazine rack next to the toilet and leave it there. Instead, you'll be proud to read it in the living room and bedroom, or, better yet, in the park, on the train, and in the coffee shop.

In his Environmental Design classic *The Bathroom* (1976), Alexander Kira notes the tendency to label any book that discusses elimination as "humor." This habit, like relegating such books to the bathroom, demonstrates the same anal-repressive need to compartmentalize and push aside our natures. Bodily functions can certainly be funny (although I think attempting humor by simply mentioning or depicting them is pretty stupid), but amusement isn't the only positive or interesting attribute they possess, and again, I think

that if we changed our outlook so as not to automatically put bodily functions in the domain of humor alone, we'd be better off. Humor often plays off things that make us uncomfortable or disturb us. We shouldn't be so uncomfortable.

Another aspect of scatological repression is its link to the middle class. In *Let Us Now Praise Famous Men* (1941), James Agee discusses "the middle-class American worship of sterility and worship-fear of its own excrement," suggesting that in this country at least, middle-class people are more anal than their lower- or upper-class compatriots. As a result, scatological themes appear much more often in Low Comedy and High Art than in mainstream cultural fare. Toilet jokes appeal to earthy folk who just plain get a kick out of them, and to intellectuals and bohemians who besides getting a kick out of them, also relish the added bonus of knowing that liking such material distinguishes them from the uptight, unhip middle class, and allies them with the "common people" they idealize and pseudo-emulate. Meanwhile, the middle class believes it proper to view such jokes as offensive. Similarly, Milan Kundera explains in *The Unbearable Lightness of Being* (1984) that kitsch, which contemptuous highbrows have always associated with the middle class, is entirely based on the denial of shit. The art of the middle class, he argues, is the art of anal repression.

Part of being repelled by our excretions probably derives from innate, health-preserving instincts that guard us from infection. But as with any of our other instincts (such as those relating to reproduction), the area where these innate individual inclinations meet and interact with the rational and society-building parts of our natures, is a fascinating tide-pool spawning many convoluted rationalizations and involved codes of conduct relating to essentially irrational behaviors. That's what makes the subject such a kick.

I found a lot of information about bodily functions at the library, but little of it explained how people today deal with the things in their daily lives. For this information, I conducted my own survey that asked people detailed questions about

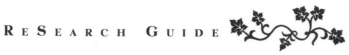

their personal hygiene habits. I got most of my "subjects" by standing out in the main plaza of the U.C. Berkeley campus with a bunch of questionnaires, pens, and dollar bills. Calling out to passers-by that they could earn a dollar by simply filling out a questionnaire quickly attracted willing people, although some of them declined to participate once I told them what the survey was about or after they leafed through the questionnaire. The survey participants, like people in general, seemed genuinely interested in their bodily functions, but because of old and destructive taboos, the subject is still seldom publicly discussed or written about. Other subjects participated through the Internet; I announced the survey on the newsgroups *rec.humor* and *alt.tasteless* and received responses from as far away as England. (Similarly, I researched the "Bodily Functions In the Cinema" chapter by posting to the newsgroup *rec.arts.movies*, and the "Urination with Genital Piercings" chapter by posting to *rec.arts.bodyart.)* The last chapter reprints the final version of the questionnaire and discusses more fully how I conducted the survey.

Three final comments: First, I deliberately deemphasized bodily fluids from the reproductive systems, not because they aren't interesting—menstrual blood is the most significant of all, culturally—but because I think sexual functioning gets plenty of press already. Second, I didn't cover disease. Fear already obscures our perception of bodily fluids, and many in the media have reacted to AIDS by adding even more irrational fear. I wanted to present a sunnier view by emphasizing health. Finally, much of this book questions attitudes and actions perpetuated by the dominant Western religious traditions but I believe that it is possible for an individual to adhere to any one of them in a thoughtful, positive, and enriching way.

Paul Spinrad, San Francisco, 1994

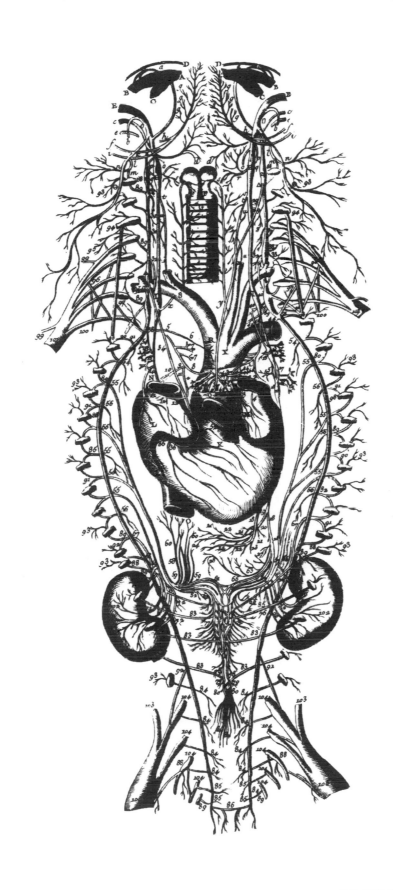

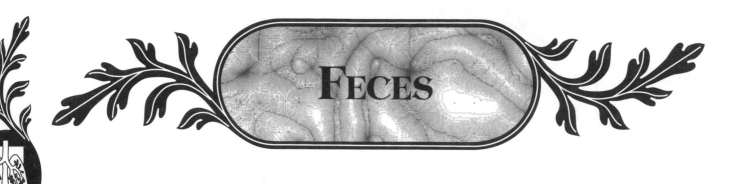

FECES

Feces

Doo doo, doody, dooty, turd, excrement, ca-ca, number two, shit, crap, log, stool, bowel movement, B.M., poop, poo-poo, ordure, pedung, night soil, dreck, sir-reverence, Zibethum Occidentalis (when prescribed as a medication), dingleberries (when adhering to anal hairs)

Animal Droppings

Dung, livestock manure, deer fewmets, cattle tath, otter spraints, cow bodewash, cow flop, sea fowl/bat guano, earthworm wormcast, hare crotiles, boar lesses, fox billitting, hawk mutes, dog scumber, game spoor, boar friants, badger werderobe, fox waggying

Defecate

Pinch a loaf, take a dump, roll a log, lose some weight, spend a dime, power dump, heave a havana, drop a load, launch a torpedo, make fudge, big job, cast your pellet, do your duty, evacuate, grunt, cover your feet, drop a spike

Fecal Prefixes

Scato-, copro-

Diarrhea

The (Hershey) squirts, Montezuma's revenge, ride the porcelain Honda, Aztec two-step, touristas

The most significant body product of them all, symbolizing the entire class, is feces. Its influence covers history, religion, agriculture, psychology, social history, anthropology, medicine, literature, the arts, architecture, design, and many other fields. Yet many of us know less about our own waste products than we do about space travel. We don't know shit.

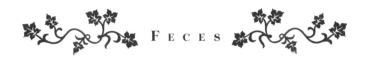

People, Places, and Pinching (Survey)

Defecation Section

Ever pinch a loaf so big that it stuck out of the water?

Most men surveyed say they have done this; most women say they have not. The total percentages are 46% Yes and 31% No. 6% answer that they aren't sure, one of them commenting, "I don't have eyes in that end of me."

Several of the big loaf pinchers temper their responses with modesty. Four Yes respondents, for example, ascribe the occurrence to small bowls or low water levels. A 31-year-old student humbly (or with false modesty) adds to his answer, "Not so much—only an inch or two." Others, however, openly boast, with answers such as, "Yes—dark, hard, well-formed 18-inch (smooth)," "Yeah—longer than the toilet bowl," and "I've even clogged the toilet." Still others state or imply that it happens to them often, writing, "Many times," "Every other day," "Of course," and "Dry dock? You bet!"

One woman relates that during childhood, her mother liked to check the size of her stools and praised her for the larger ones. Even more positive reinforcement came "when we could poop and pee at the same time. It was always an exciting event filled with praise. 'Great! Congratulations!'"

"No" responses exhibit a variety of feelings, including envy ("No, wish I could," "Never had the pleasure"), disgust ("Sick—no"), and disbelief ("Ahem, yeah right."). Finally, one special case answers, "Not except for floaters."

Ever wipe with leaves? Dirt? Your hand? Paper money?

The clear leader among the TP substitutes mentioned here is leaves. An even 50% say they've wiped with leaves, far surpassing the 8% who say they've used their hands, the second place answer. Only 2% say they've used dirt or paper money.

Three people state that they used leaves while camping. Another leaf-wiper adds that moss is better. A 29-year-old who claims to like the outdoors says he used leaves while on his newspaper route. A 17-year-old with solid values answers, "With leaves! Money is too gross."

The two money-wipers have different attitudes. The older one, a 41-year-old, answers, "Money (in Brazil, where it's worthless)." The younger, a 20-year-old who describes himself as a "drug advocate" explains, "Yes—once when I was drunk and pissed at the system." Meanwhile, a young man who works as a telemarketer answers, "No—but there's an idea." A 24-year-old sports promoter gives the compound answer, "Yes. No. Yuck. I wish I was that rich."

Several participants mention other wipes they've used. A programmer writes, "No. No. No. No, but I have used notebook paper, a newspaper, a sock, a bandanna, a flannel shirt." Other items mentioned include pine cones, rocks, paper toilet seat covers, and snow. Finally, one 37-year-old smarty jokes, "No, I always use little white rabbits and hot water."

Do you crumple your toilet paper, fold it, or wrap it?

42% fold, 33% crumple, 8% say they do a little of both, 6% wrap it around, and 3% say it depends on their mood or on the type of paper. Women favor crumpling and wrapping and men favor folding, but the correlation is weak.

Some respondents seem to associate folding with, well, anality. An 18-year-old folder adds, "I'm neat." A 27-year-old explains, "Usually fold, crumple when rushed." A young woman of 20 answers, "Crumple. But if I'm feeling compulsive, I fold." A young man writes, "Fold. It cleans better."

A 30-year-old programmer, on the other hand, responds, "Crumple—what kind of weirdo would fold it?" A grad student, 25, announces, "I'm a crumpler."

Finally, a teenage boy answers, "Toss it in the toilet as is."

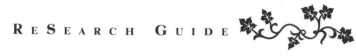

About how many squares do you tear off at once? About how many wipes do you get per tear? About how many tears will take care of your average loaf?

Several people give answers like "depends," "a lot," or "more than average," but most participants supply numbers or number ranges. The results? Squares per tear: range 2-20, mean 5.90, median 5, mode 4. Wipes per tear: range 1-10, mean 2.0, median 1.5, mode 2. Tears per loaf: range 1-12, mean 3.23, median and mode 3.

Where both squares/tear and tears/loaf were supplied, I multiplied to produce squares per loaf. Results: range 8-55, mean 17.94, median 15, modes at 10 and 20.

A 20-year-old student tops the list on squares per tear with 20. He gets three wipes per tear and usually tears only once per visit, yielding a near-average 20 squares total usage. Elsewhere he explains that he defecates once a day and wraps his toilet paper around his hand 4-6 times to get the proper amount.

Another male student, 24, leads the pack in wipes per tear, squeezing ten of them out of just three squares. He does this twice for each dump, on average, using only six squares total — the lowest squares/loaf number among the men. He pinches once daily, folds his paper, and uses the back-and-forth method of wiping.

The most common wipe per tear count is two, but one-per-tear runs close behind. One vocal defendant of this sizable minority explains, "One wipe per, as I don't care to shove something covered with shit back up my butt, and I find the idea of searching for a clean spot even more revolting." Another asks, "Who wants to wipe with a shitty wad of T.P.?"

Average tears/loaf range from one to twelve, the twelve at the high end being supplied by a 29-year-old man who elsewhere says that he moistens his toilet paper "if my ass is raw." Five people say they typically tear only once per visit. Two of them say they look at the paper after a wipe, while the other three say they look "sometimes." One single-tearer, a graduate student in Oceanic Engineering who nevertheless doesn't seem to be much of a problem-solver, answers in full, "Roughly two feet. One wipe, one tear, but ALWAYS inadequate."

The two respondents who use the least total paper are two of the single-tear people, young women who both tear off four sheets, wipe twice, looking "sometimes," and are done with it. At the other extreme sits a 31-year-old woman who typically uses up five or six crumpled ten-square lengths of paper, wiping once or twice with each.

A 25-year-old explains that he pulls off lots of paper in public restrooms with "mongo rolls." Elsewhere, he limits himself to four squares per tear. Finally, a 31-year-old male student who uses a modest 10.5 squares per loaf, nevertheless excuses himself with, "I have a hairy butt."

Do you wipe front to back (i.e. bottom to top), back to front, or just back and forth? Do you reach around behind your back or reach back through between your legs?

44% say they wipe front to back from around behind their backs. 11% say they wipe back to front between their legs. 6% go back to front from behind their backs, and 4%, all women, go front to back between their legs. 2% say they go back and forth (!) from behind their backs.

Several respondents answer incompletely. 11% just say they go front to back, 3% simply say they go back to front, and 2% say they go back and forth, all without giving their approaches. Similarly, 2% just say they go around back, and one just answers "side from right." These answers were not summed into the totals above.

Of the 21 people who go back to front, only four are women, probably because, as one Women's Studies major points out, going back to front causes vaginal infections. This concern may have combined with women's from-the-front urine blotting habits to yield the uniquely female between-the-legs, front-to-back solution used by 4% of the sample.

Several front-to-back people add that they sometimes utilize back-to-front or back-and-forth action for the messier ones. But some people vary their technique for other reasons. One young

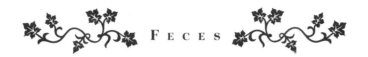

woman writes, "It depends on how I feel that day."

Do you look at the paper after a wipe?

60%, mostly men, say they do and 14%, mostly women, say they do not. Another 16% say they do it sometimes, and 1% say they do it only if they're getting close to their periods.

Twelve respondents who say they look ask questions like, "How else do you know if you're finished?," or ·explain that they do it to judge the status of their cleaning. Six respondents answer with "Of course." Other comments by respondents who answer Yes include, "Most definitely. Determines one's health," "It's half the fun to see what it looks like," "That's the pudding after dinner," and, more apologetically, "It's kind of hard not to if it's in your hand."

Meanwhile, one teen who says she does not look answers, "NEVER—I'd ·throw up."

Do you stand to wipe or remain seated and lean over?

72 of the 106 respondents were asked this question. Of that group, 58%, mostly women, say they remain seated, while 25%, mostly men, say they stand. 3% say they squat or "semi-stand," 1% say they bend slightly, and 1% say they do both: "Usually remain seated unless it's a heavy job."

Do you like to watch it go down after a flush?

Only 46 questionnaires contained this question. Of those respondents, 43% say they don't, 28% say they do, 13% say they sometimes do, and 7% explain that they watch to confirm a complete flush. One young man explains, "I do generally at home, not a strong flush. I wouldn't say I 'like to.' " Meanwhile, a middle-aged man answers, "50%," while a young woman writes, "I don't care really."

Ever moisten the paper for improved cleaning ability? How?

Most respondents, 62%, answer No. Some give reasons: "No way, butt-rash city," "No—it just gets all shredded," "I don't need to." Others share different solutions: "I wash it off in the bathtub

sometimes," "Sometimes I don't wipe, I just jump in the shower." Still others express unfamiliarity: "No, what a strange idea," "No—good idea." One 21-year-old woman answers, "No, but my mom does."

The 25% who say they sometimes moisten the paper give conditions as well as methods for this action. One man, the tears-per-loaf recordholder in the sample, moistens only when his "ass is raw." Others do it only "after a bad one (i.e. dingleberry day)" or "after radical diarrhea."

Moistening methods vary, but by far the most popular, with over half the moistener vote, is using water from the faucet. Several people use spittle, a few just state they use water without naming the source, two dip into the toilet after flushing, and a 20-year-old student explains, "Sometimes use faucet or own urine-drops from dick."

Others branch out into new materials. A 39-year-old woman uses water on paper towels, and a 22-year-old man mentions "moist wipes" (foil-wrapped disposable moist towelettes).

Does eating highly-spiced foods affect your loaves the next day?

42% say it does, 27% say it doesn't, 8% don't know, 7% say they haven't noticed it, 4% say it happens occasionally, 1% answer "probably," and 1% answer "only once."

Fourteen respondents mention a burning sensation ("jaloproctosis" is the newly-coined medical term), with answers such as "Yes—burn city" and "Stagg Chili leaves burning logs." Three more mention a general pain or stinging with words that carry no sense of combustion, like the sports promoter who answers, "Sometimes it makes my butthole sting after the loaf is out, but the loaf doesn't seem to mind."

Six people say spicy foods make their stools thinner, looser, or even "fragile," including one young man who explains, "They aren't loaves after spicy food—it's more like crepes." Another young man alludes to diarrhea with his answer: "Oh man—quesadilla salsa explosion." Other respondents report that spicy foods give their feces

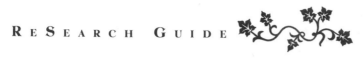

strange colors, make them smellier, and increase their size.

Meanwhile, a 38-year-old woman adds that rich foods and beer also affect her loaves, and a 20-year-old man says that grape juice gives his stools a greenish cast. Finally, an Internet respondent who describes himself as a "dirty old man" makes the inevitable pun, "How would the baker know what I have eaten and why should it affect him?"

Does drinking coffee help give you "the urge"? Smoking a cigarette?

Both activities invite Nature's Call, but coffee-drinking, the one more popular with the sample group, seems to do it more. 37% say coffee does help, as opposed to 9% who say it doesn't. Cigarette smoking, on the other hand, gets 14% Yes and 14% No.

Participants mention other effects of coffee-drinking, including diarrhea. "[Too much] coffee gives me the Hershey squirts," writes one young man. Other respondents say that colas, cafe mochas, and hot chocolate, three other caffeine-containing beverages, prompt them to defecate. Writes one young woman, "Hot chocolate makes me doo doo."

Two respondents provide other laxative hints. A young man of 20 shares, "Finger up the ass does the trick." Another young man, a grad student of 25, writes, "The best laxative I have yet to find is going into a bookstore to browse. Painful sphincter-clenching ensues within minutes." (In *Room Temperature*, Nicholson Baker claims that libraries have a similar effect.)

Would you consider yourself "regular"? How many loaves do you pinch per day? At what times?

Nearly half the sample, 49%, consider themselves regular. 15% do not, 5% say they are sometimes or usually regular, and 3% don't know. Some respondents suggest clockwork regularity in answering the question's third part, like the 24-year-old student who writes, "9:15 AM (after 1st cup of coffee)," or the geologist who answers, "7 AM, 4 PM." Various irregular respondents, meanwhile, lament their fate, like the grad student who answers, "No, unfortunately, 1/2, morning." Others celebrate it, like the young Briton who says he's "quite irregular."

Respondents' defecation frequencies range from once every two to three days, to five times daily. The average is 1.67 per day, the mean is 1.5, and the most frequent response, supplied by well over one-third of respondents who stated frequencies, is once daily. All of those who claim to defecate four or more times per day are males. One, a 25-year-old programmer, says elsewhere that he stopped eating high-fiber cereals because they made his stools too frequent. Another, a 27-year-old lawyer, eats oat bran cereal "often" and says that the longest he has ever gone without pinching a loaf is one-and-a-half days. A 31-year-old student who defecates four to five times per day (and "sometimes more") says the longest he has gone without a bowel movement is "about a day." Meanwhile, a 26-year-old software methodologist who ordinarily defecates once or twice a day says that if he's nervous or sick he might go "as many as eight to ten" times per day.

Morning is the most popular time to defecate, mentioned by 28% of the sample. Night and afternoon net 11% each, no particular time/whenever necessary nets 10%, and evening nets 9%. Many respondents also say they like to visit the toilet after meals, especially after lunch, or, as one 20-year-old computer programmer puts it, "After lunch (at work so that I can be paid $7.75 an hour to dump)."

Ever see kernels of corn in your loaves? Peanuts? Tomato seeds? Other distinguishable objects?

45% say they've observed corn, 19% say they've spotted peanuts, and 8% say they've detected tomato seeds. One man puns, "I'm a cornucopia." Meanwhile, 14% simply answer Yes, or as another punster puts it, "Of coarse," and 6% echo the sentiments of the young man who writes, "No. I guess I don't look at my doody carefully."

Responding to the last part of the question,

participants list a second-harvest bounty which includes leafy green vegetables (lettuce, spinach, and "dark leaves"), seeds (fruit seeds, caraway seeds, melon seeds, sunflower seeds and seed husks, watermelon seeds, kidney beans, and "rice?"), keratinous materials (shrimp shells and fish scales), other organic matter (tomato skin, carrots, peach skin, and asparagus fibers), and even inorganic materials (tiny rocks, marbles, pennies, and LEGO® pieces). Two respondents also cite foods that have reddened their stools: watermelon and beets (Tom Robbins mentions this characteristic of beets in *Jitterbug Perfume*).

Do you eat a breakfast cereal? A high-fiber variety? Are you pleased with its effect on your stool?

45% say they eat cereal, and another 7% say they sometimes do. 27% say they eat a high-fiber cereal, 9% say they do not, and 10% say they vary their breakfast. 21% say they're pleased, as opposed to only 2% who say they're not. Meanwhile, 25%, including some who don't eat high-fiber breakfast cereals, say that they haven't noticed any effect or that fiber doesn't affect them.

The "we're pleased" group expresses warmth, debt, and quiet power with answers such as, "Yes, very much, thank you" and "very pleased." A young man of 26 answers, "Yes. Yes. Yes!!!" An older man, 37, writes, "Yes. Yes. You bet!" A 30-year-old male programmer elaborates, "Sometimes. Yes. Oh, definitely. I find that Raisin Bran or some such produces huge, loose, bowl-filling, foul-smelling fecal masses, and a more satisfying 'empty' feeling after a dump." A 47-year-old machinist who says he finds bodily functions "enjoyable if not outright pleasurable," brings up another factor: "Yes, and it makes for some KILLER farts, especially when topped with bananas."

Meanwhile, a 24-year-old architecture student laments, "Cracklin' Oat Bran used to give me really nice ones, but I seem to have developed a tolerance." Similarly, a 22-year-old student complains, "It should do more than it does. I want Colon Blow!" Two other respondents, on the

other hand, find high-fiber cereal overly effective, saying they stopped eating it because it made them defecate more frequently than they preferred.

The wet-blanket attitude of some of the less fecally-aware of the survey's participants is well captured by the 20-year-old programmer who writes, "I eat cereal because it tastes okay in the morning. I don't notice its effect."

Do you ever avoid any food or any class of food because you don't like the effect it has on your loaves?

59% say they don't, 25% say they do, and 2% just say they haven't thought about it.

Respondents who don't avoid foods show confidence in their priorities with answers like, "No way" and "No, I'll eat fuckin' near anything." But the food-avoiding set must weigh issues of constipation, diarrhea, farting, and social interaction as well as food appeal during their complex determinations.

Several people single beans out—refried beans in burritos, homemade beans, black bean soup, or just beans in general. One woman writes, "Sometimes I don't eat beans before I'll see people." A man warns, "Avoid Black Bean Soup! I ate one bowl of this at a friend's, and I spent the next four days farting and shitting like never before."

Others mention spicy or pungent foods or cuisines, including onions, garlic, hot peppers, bay leaves, Mexican food, Chinese food, and spicy foods in general. One 25-year-old man writes, "Sometimes I think twice about spicy food, but I usually go for it anyway."

One young woman says sugary foods give her diarrhea. A 37-year-old man writes, "You bet! Pizza makes ball turds." A woman of 20 avoids dairy products because of Irritable Bowel Syndrome. A man of 30 simply says that excess meat or dairy has "a bad effect." Meanwhile, a 39-year-old woman generalizes that "Cheese is binding and constipation is painful," leaving the conclusion as an exercise for the reader.

Participants also make mention of Lite Beer,

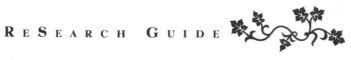

Shaeffer beer, pizza, Ex-Lax, prunes, most fast foods (especially Burger King's "BK Broilers"), "sausage from the University pizza place," and, understandably, parasites.

Are you reluctant to pinch a loaf away from home? What's the most uncomfortable place you've ever had to pinch a loaf?

37%, mostly men, say they are not reluctant to pinch one away from home, while 25%, mostly women, say they are. One young man says he only defecates at home and never at work, while another remarks, "If I gotta go, I gotta go." 5% more say they only balk if the unfamiliar facilities are dirty or otherwise off-putting.

Survey participants clearly dislike moving their bowels out of doors. 8% give the woods of the forest as the most uncomfortable place they've pinched. Another 7% specify parks, fields, hills, or "the wild." 2% mention doing it in bushes. Another 2%, by the side of the road. Others remember leaning over poison ivy and over rocks. A 37-year-old man recalls being swarmed by insects in the Finnish tundra. A younger man remembers trying to relieve himself roadside at the age of seven, losing his balance, and falling down a short slope. A woman recalls hiding inside her poncho while defecating by the road in treeless, rockless country above the timber line.

6% mention porta-potties or outhouses, often in wilderness areas. One 22-year-old remarks, "Portapotties scare me." A 20-year-old recalls "an isolated outhouse with splinters, and the [excrement] level was six inches from the top." Another 4% mention latrine tents or long drops used on camping trips.

5% say they've been most uncomfortable at the houses or apartments of dates, girlfriends, or boyfriends. Another 2% mention other people's homes in general. One young man recalls, "Once I did a big loud spray-mist shit in a bathroom while about three girls waited outside the door."

7% mention stalls in public restrooms. One young man recalls "the same McDonald's bathroom stall that my prom date had already yakked in." 3% mention public facilities that lacked stalls,

including a young man who recalls "Sitting in the *crowded* bathroom at the Stud [a men's bar] in San Francisco. Toilet just out there." A young woman recalls a public restroom "without stalls—just a row of toilets." On the other side of the coin, however, a 25-year-old writes, "Actually, I kind of like public restrooms if they're clean and have good graffiti."

3% say the worst place they've defecated is in their pants. One young woman recalls having soiled herself in a library in fifth grade and that she wasn't allowed to sit down in the car on the way home.

Other difficult places of easement include bars and clubs; a high-school bathroom; a Turkish toilet in Pamplona, Spain; a hospital bedpan; a boat; a car; Mexico; a fancy restaurant; an airplane; and a "Rainbow Gathering." Respondents also mention three more general situations: during meetings, when the phone rings, and "when you have gas in a bathroom near a lot of stoned people."

Do you fear "toilet water splash-back"? Do you like it?

30%, mostly women, write that they fear splash-back, while 9%, all but one of them men, say they like it. Meanwhile, 38% say they don't fear it and/or don't like it either. 2% indicate that they have both reactions at once, a feeling well described by a 26-year-old software engineer who writes, "I fear it and like it (it feels good, but . . .)."

Negative reactions vary. 4% say they "hate" toilet water splash-back. Others question whether the word "fear" best describes their feelings. A teenage girl writes, ambiguously, "Yes, a lot. Fear isn't the word for it." Another young woman remarks, "Fear is a strong word." An older man writes, "Always. Never. Once I pooped in an *outhouse* and got splash-back! Yuck!!!!" A cautious 22-year-old answers, "To a certain extent, yes." The 27-year-old man who recalls having once urinated off a cliff "whilst" thinking of the Brontë sisters explains, "Fear would be a primitive response . . . . Can't say I exactly cotton to it." A 20-year-old man writes, "Hell yes, especially when I've already pissed in it." Another explains,

"I hate it if it gets on my butt cheeks, but otherwise it's okay." Finally, a young woman of 21 answers, "Yes. No, I don't like it 'cause all the shit goes on my butt."

On the other side of the fence stand people who feel that, "It's kinda refreshing," "It's a wonderful thing," "[It's] not bad, kinda nice really," "[It] improves cleaning," and even, "No—real men enjoy splash-back." 3% say they sometimes fear it, or only fear it in unfamiliar or dirty bathrooms.

Two respondents mention that they put toilet paper in the water beforehand in order to avoid the splash. Others, however, seem ignorant of this phenomenon. A computer scientist in his late thirties writes, "No, there is quite a distance between my bottom and the surface." An upbeat 18-year-old woman remarks, "I've never had the luck to experience it!"

Finally, 7% of respondents say they accept the phenomenon, live with it, or are indifferent to it. One describes his feelings as, "Indifferent, almost ataraxic," which means that his reaction to toilet water splash-back is "almost" like the tranquil state of mind the Skeptic philosophers sought through examining and understanding all the diverse and contradictory viewpoints on a matter and not judging one to be superior to any others.

Are you a world traveler? How have you found foreign types of toilets to be?

Only 22% of the sample characterize themselves as world travelers, but many who don't make relevant comments nevertheless. Respondents note "shelf" toilets in Austria, Germany, and Eastern Europe, "Turkish" or "squat" toilets in Italy, China, Greece, Vietnam, and the Arab world, toilets with no seats in the Dominican Republic, and "normal" toilets in the UK, New Zealand, France, Italy, Germany, and Mexico. They also remark that they have disliked, for various reasons, toilets in Guatemala, Mexico, India, China, Germany, and Southern Europe.

Reactions vary. 9% say they've found foreign toilets to be familiar enough and perfectly fine. 8% say they're sometimes dirty or disgusting. Another 5% have found them displeasing or in-

ferior for reasons unstated. 3% have observed heavier toilet paper, 2% say they use less water, and various others say they're cleaner, more efficient, more primitive, too public, and, from a 31-year-old woman baker/student/fine artist, "Dirty, but blessedly generic (no 'men' or 'women' status)."

On squat toilets, participants assume a variety of stances. A middle-aged machinist answers, "Only been to 'Nam. Squat toilets in 'Nam were a tad strange at first, but I grew to prefer them." A younger man writes, "I'm in love with the Italian holes (a.k.a. squat 'n' shoot)." Another simply finds squat holes "amusing." Meanwhile, a 25-year-old comments, "I hate 'starter blocks,'" accompanying his text with a stick figure illustration. One young observer writes, "Greek hole-in-the-ground types give you the 'shitter's thighs,' i.e. enlarged quadriceps. Eastern European 'shelf toilets' seem not to actually flush, and display your efforts prominently."

No one liked the "inspection shelf" type of toilet. No respondent mentioned this, but from other sources I'm told that lining the shelf with paper before defecating prevents the stool from leaving the characteristic streak marks.

One young woman remarks that she prefers bidets to toilet paper. Another writes that "the French use sandpaper." A young Internet respondent from an unidentified country (my guess is it's England, but I detached message headers upon receipt to assure anonymity), answers, "Only New Zealand and USA. Hate USA toilets . . . they make the shit really float up and look at you (with the water being so close to your backside)." A none-too-tolerant 30-year-old woman writes, "In Latin America they are disgusting—people are pigs." Finally, an 18-year-old male student and self-described "friend to the universe" writes, "No seats. Interesting institutional/psychological dynamic connections."

What's your "record" for how long you've gone without pinching a loaf? Were you traveling then?

The most common quantitative answer here

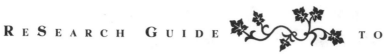

(57% give actual numbers) is 3 days and the median answer is 3.5 days, but two astounding statistical outliers, a 24-year-old man who didn't shit for two weeks while traveling and a 31-year-old woman who as a child did not defecate for an entire three-week session of summer camp, help raise the average constipation interval up to 4.47 days. At the opposite end of the curve, two respondents say their record is one day. One, a 31-year-old man, normally defecates 4-5 times daily, while the other, a woman of the same age, goes 2-3 times daily and understandably considers herself "regular." Meanwhile, 14% say they don't know or haven't counted, and several others give answers such as, "a few days," "not long at all," "a long time," and "days."

24% say they were indeed traveling at the time, as opposed to 8% who say they were not, but others give their own circumstances, which include skiing, "fear of porta-potties," at summer camp, while camping, as a child, while fasting, while on a fruit diet, during survival training (with no solid food), after knee surgery, while in New York, and while in Kansas.

What Is A Loaf?

If you've vomited both right after, and a long interval after, a meal; and if you've had diarrhea and looser-than-average stools; then, if you were paying any attention at all, you probably have a fairly accurate qualitative sense of the changes the contents of our digestive tracts go through on their downward journey. Vomit from immediately after a meal is chunkier and less homogenous than more "mature" vomit, and diarrhea's severity, the degree to which it is from our bodies untimely wrought, correlates with its liquidity. As this suggests, our food gets churned up with digestive juices into a blended liquid, and then the nutrient-filled liquid part is gradually removed, yielding solid waste. This much we know.

The average healthy adult stool weighs approximately one-quarter to one-half pound, and measures from four to eight inches in length and one-half to one-and-one-half inches in width. 65% of it is water, 5-10% is nitrogen, 10-20% are soluble substances, and another 10-20% are ash.

These statistics describe the texture and size of feces but not its color, as those who eat only dairy products are quick to point out. Normal feces are always a shade of brown, because contrary to common understanding, the digestive tract not only accomodates food and digestive juices, but also serves as a dumping ground for bodily wastes generated elsewhere, most relevantly bilirubin, a yellow by-product of the decomposition of old red blood cells, and also a close chemical relative of hemoglobin. The liver adds bilirubin to bile, the fat-digesting liquid it secretes via the gall-bladder into the beginning of the small intestine. But bilirubin has no known digestive function of its own; it's just along for the ride, and bile provides a convenient escape route.

The helpful bacteria in the small intestine which aid digestion also convert bilirubin into hydrobilirubin, or urobilin, a yellow-brown pigment also present in urine. In the lower intestines, the stool-to-be undergoes a drying-out and solidifying process which concentrates the yellow-brown color, yielding a more familiar darker-brown. It's interesting to note that despite the color's prevalence, no national flag includes a field of brown and many languages, including ancient Greek and ancient Chinese, even lack a word for it.

The bacterial transformation of yellow bilirubin to brown urobilin explains why meconium, the feces excreted by fetuses and newborns, is yellow; the lower digestive tract of the newborn has not yet been populated by the normally-resident bacteria. One professor at Cornell's School of Veterinary Medicine dramatically demonstrated the absolute sterility of meconium by eating a spoonful scooped from the colon of a dissected fetal calf in front of his class!

Like most natural processes, digestion is not completely efficient. Humans defecate about one-quarter of the protein present in rice and potatoes and 40% of the protein in corn meal. In addition, in a process known as *refection*, intestinal bacteria generate nutrients below the point where the body can absorb them, and these are excreted as well. As a result, feces can actually provide a lot of nutrition. Humans do not take advantage of feces as a nutritional source, for various reasons, but many (and perhaps most) other one-stomached animals regularly do, including rabbits, dogs, pigs, mice, chickens, guinea pigs, and rats. Rats probably top the list as the most voracious consumers of their own feces, eating about half of their one-time-through feces under normal dietary conditions, and sometimes all of their feces under a vitamin-deficient diet. Experiments involving rats in wire-screen cages who have been fitted with "tail cups" to prevent coprophagy have resulted in severe malnutrition. The rat's strong coprophagic nature was cited as a factor early in this century when scientists first began using them for experiments, and this should still be considered and accounted for in any experiments in which rats are being fed.

Even if you haven't paid attention when you've vomited or suffered diarrhea, you probably have some idea of how the food you eat affects your stools. An array of fecal attributes, including size, color, and texture, are under your creative control when you choose what you eat and how you live. These attributes are:

Size: Obviously, absolute food intake correlates with stool size. Food type matters as well, with vegetables, bran, and other sources of water-retaining fiber contributing to big, healthy loaves, and highly concentrated, rich, fatty foods such as meat, eggs, cheese, and buttered white bread generating small, slow-moving ones. More complete cooking and chewing reduce size as well, but not for the same reasons as do meat, et al; cooking and chewing make the job of the rest of the tract (extracting nutrients) easier and more thorough, while meat simply gums up the works. The size has to do with water content, which the large intestine reduces as a final step, so the overdue products of constipation tend to be small. The largest stools of all are the waterlogged, whole-intestine wonders that follow enemas, with the record weighing-in at 20 kilograms, the weight

of an average first-grader (the comparison brings up another fact, that per body weight, children's stools are larger than adults'). Size and water content are closely related to a second characteristic:

Density: Regular users of flush toilets of non-German manufacture know that feces are usually denser than water, although "floaters" are not unheard of, particularly among vegetarians and people whose intestines produce a lot of methane (intestinal methane production is an inherited trait associated with more-frequent farting). Bubbles aside, density correlates inversely with water content, making the smaller, less healthy, often overdue, animal-origin stools harder and heavier than those of predominantly vegetable origin.

Texture: This reflects density: lower density, softer texture. Undigested inclusions, such as corn kernels and tomato and pepper seeds, can play an ancillary role. Seeds can pass through the digestive tract with remarkably little damage, as evidenced by the remarks of a farmer at the 11 March 1939 meeting of the Northeastern Branch of the Institute of Sewage Purification in England, as cited by Reginald Reynolds (in *Cleanliness and Godliness*, 1941), who praised sewage sludge for providing him with excellent tomato plants without the necessity of sowing seeds.

Shape: [I frequently refer to the contrast between high-fiber stools and the smaller, meat- and dairy-diet types, and for brevity, I'll label the first type "G" and the second type "NG."] Type G loaves taper fairly uniformly, often breaking apart while in motion. NG loaves, however, generally stay in one piece and have bumps and ridges resulting from their long motionless tenures against wrinkles in the interior of the large intestine. Scybala, small balls of feces which often cluster together to form another characteristic shape of the NG stool, also form in the wrinkled recesses of the colon when things aren't moving along as quickly as they should. It's unfortunate that this pebble-cluster shape, arguably the most visually interesting of all, is not associated with intestinal health.

Color: G loaves tend toward a lighter yellowish-brown, while NG loaves are a darker brown

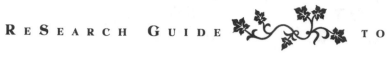

or even, following a meal of blood sausages or blood puddings, black. Large quantities of red meat will darken the stool considerably. In addition, certain special foods or chemical agents can produce other shades. For some, eating beets results in a reddish hue. Milk adds a yellowish accent, and rhubarb can add a stronger yellow. Consuming Methylene Blue, a chemical used as a bacteriological stain and as an antidote for cyanide poisoning, will create a stool that turns blue-green with exposure to air. Eating the metallic element Bismuth will turn the stool dark green or black. Senna, a flowering plant used as a cathartic; gamboge, a brownish tree resin used as a yellow pigment; and santonin, an anthelmintic found in wormwood; will make yellow. Kino, a reddish tree resin, will make bright red. Large amounts of iron will make dark gray, after air exposure. Hematoxylin, a dye chemical extracted from logwood, a tropical American tree, will make violet or reddish-violet. Calomel, a mercury compound used as a purgative, produces green, but a slightly greenish cast can result from the ingestion of large quantities of blackberries or huckleberries. Senna and wormwood are available at most herbal/botanical stores. Scientific supply stores carry bismuth and Methylene Blue. Author does not condone and accepts no responsibility for any individual's ingestion of any substance here discussed.

Odor: A stool's unique odor, like that of a fart, primarily derives from volatile chemicals produced by intestinal bacteria breaking down food's more chemically-complex nutrients; subsequently, diet and intestinal health are the main variables affecting odor. Feces produced while fasting, composed largely of urobilin and other nonfood body wastes, have little or no odor, while the stools of alcoholics, whose drinking habits are tough on intestinal flora, are extra-smelly. To most people, feces' potential variety of chemicals and chemical ratios merely means that loaves have characteristic smells, but forensic scientists have used feces' unique chemical signatures to help track and catch criminals.

Wiping Through History (And Around the World)

Before the dawn of civilization, sticks and stones were almost certainly among the first objects used as tools for tasks as diverse as cracking nuts, digging roots, and killing strangers, but anthropologists might also consider their use in another very old task: ass-wiping. Animals don't usually wipe themselves, but humans are different; their varied and unpredictable, omnivorous diet means their digestion can't sufficiently specialize to produce a "clean one" every time. Consequently, humans possessed of ingenuity, dexterity, and an occasional interest in cleanliness will come up with handy solutions.

Simple "found" objects comprised the earliest wipes, many of which still enjoy popularity today. These include sticks, stones, leaves, dry bones, hay, and shells. Mussel shells, common enough and certainly conveniently sized and shaped, were a popular wipe in coastal areas in this country until the ascendancy of toilet paper around 1900. Hawaiians used coconut husks. Aristophanes wrote that the rich used leeks. Medieval monks used pottery shards and cloth fragments. The middle classes in France during the 1600's used unspun hemp. Meanwhile, ladies of the court of Louis XIV used wool and even lace.

Of course, the simplest wipe, still one of the best and most popular, is the hand, traditionally the left hand, which can't really count as a "tool," although if you stretch it, you could consider as the enabling tool the water or earth used to cleanse the hand afterwards.

Left-hand wiping is common in India and the Arab world, and many people there consider the Western practice of using paper and the right hand disgusting. How can dry paper cleanse? And to an extent, they're right. Smearing with dry paper, no matter how absorbent, will leave a residue.

The objection to using the right hand stems from the convention of eating with the right hand

and wiping with the left. For this reason, many cultures traditionally consider using the left hand to pass food to someone at the table as an insult.

Islamic tradition prescribes another way of cleaning up: wipe with stones or clods of earth, rinse with water, and then dry with a linen cloth. Pious men carry clods of earth in their turbans and small pitchers of water for this purpose, and because they believe urine makes all it touches impure, they traditionally blot the end of the penis with pebbles, clods, or against a wall. This last method gave rise to the traditional practical joke, performed by non-Muslims living around the Eastern Mediterranean, of dusting outdoor walls at penis level with ground hot pepper. Interestingly, in *The Bathroom: Criteria for Design*, Professor Alexander Kira recommends that all men, like women, blot after urinating, as Islamic law requires.

In Ancient Rome, public toilets (and probably many private ones as well) provided a sponge attached to the end of a stick, and soaking in a bucket of brine. Seneca's Epistle No. 70 describes a German slave's committing suicide by ramming one of these sticks down his throat. Owing to its widespread use, the sponge-on-a-stick apparatus was probably as familiar to the Romans as toilet paper is to us.

If you find the image of a sponge on a stick somehow familiar, but don't think it's because of its role in ancient hygiene, you're probably remembering its mention in the accounts of Jesus's crucifixion in the Gospels of Matthew (27:48), Mark (16:36), and John (19:29).

The descriptions differ slightly, but in each of them, the crucified Jesus is surrounded by a mocking crowd, one member of which pushes a sponge on a stick, soaked in a noxious liquid (vinegar or sour wine), in his face. Immediately after this ultimate indignity, the last in a series that includes being laughed at, poked at, being forced to wear a crown of thorns, and having a sarcastic sign posted on his cross, Jesus dies.

Related details differ, but the Gospels all agree that the mob present was ridiculing Jesus. The sponge on a stick present at the Crucifixion carried scatological associations fully in keeping with this mocking tone, connotations which we have since lost in our era of *Charmin*.

Affluent Romans also wiped with wool and rosewater. The number of options increased in the Middle Ages with the advent of a curved stick to do the main part of the job, coupled with mempiria, balls of hay which applied the final polish. Widespread usage of this curved stick spawned the expression "to get hold of the wrong end of the stick," an old variation of which survives in Northern England as "to get hold of the moocky end of the stick." The excavation of an old monastery at St. Albans revealed remnants of torn-up gowns of coarse cloth placed by the privy during the Middle Ages.

During the late Middle Ages, France contributed significantly to ass-wiping, producing François Rabelais, whose books *Gargantua* and *Pantagruel* delve into the subject in great detail, and developing the bidet. Early bidets were simply small tubs atop low pedestals, but later advances in toilet technology added running water and drains, and bidets became common in France early in this century. World War I British and American soldiers first saw the fixtures in French brothels and brought back to their own countries the misconception that bidets were specifically for vaginal douching (by prostitutes especially), rather than for general perineal-anal-genital cleansing by both sexes. This perceptual error has no doubt prevented the sensible, paper-saving fixture from catching on in this country.

Colonial America had its own wipe-of-choice. Corn cobs were the leading wipe in this country until paper became the standard, and even then they remained a close second for decades. The standard privy out back had a box of cobs on the floor, and folk custom prescribed that the red cobs outnumber the white ones, the reasoning being that you start with a red one, use a white one to see if you need to continue, and then use another red one if necessary.

Daily news journals became popular during the 1700's, and as a result printed matter soon became Western Europe and America's favorite

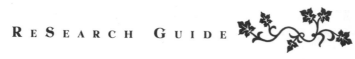

wipe. One reference to this is found in a letter from Lord Chesterfield (1694-1773) to his son (a letter which his son fortunately kept), in which he advises the young man to carry with him a cheap edition of the Latin poets, giving him something improving to read while on the toilet, as well as a good use for each finished page. Mail sorters on trains were known to use letters for this identical function. In 1906, German composer Max Reger responded to the critic Rudolph Louis in a famous letter, "I am sitting in the smallest room of my house. I have your review before me. In a moment, it will be behind me." Similar sentiments lie behind the English slang term "bumph," meaning "worthless stuff," and originating from the phrase "bum fodder."

Paper's popularity as an ass-wrotewipe inevitably caused some littering of the landscape. According to legend, when Dr. Whewell, the Master of Trinity College in Cambridge was showing Trinity to Queen Victoria, the queen asked about all the pieces of paper floating on the river Cam. Whewell replied that they were "notices that bathing is forbidden." Ignoring anachronism, the same exchange has also been attributed to Queen Victoria and Dean Jonathan Swift.

In the rural America of the late 19th Century, the main source of paper was the thick semi-annual Sears catalog, often hung up on a nail inside the privy. The catalog provided hundreds of pages of absorbent, uncoated paper, even after the concerned mother removed the "Female Undergarments" and "Personal Hygiene" sections for the benefit of the boys. Old-timers still preferred cobs, but catalog paper was the choice of a new generation, and business folk in the cities referred to America's farmlands as "the cob and catalog belt." Many country folk complained when, around the early 1930's, mail-order companies started printing their catalogs on glossy, clay-coated paper.

Paper produced specifically for wiping, toilet paper, was first produced in England in 1880. This early TP was not packaged on rolls; it consisted of individual squares stacked in boxes or strung on strings. The Victorian practice of women curling their hair by rolling it around small pieces of paper provided the convenient euphemism "curl papers" or "curling papers." In 1907 crêped paper, the forerunner of modern soft tissue, was first marketed in the U.S. The British, however, stuck with "hard tissue," and still prefer it today. Americans don't generally like British TP, but the Belgians do, and they buy a lot of British TP (marketed there as "British No. 3") for its quiet snob appeal.

The use of toilet paper caught on gradually, but just as writing paper had been used for wiping, this specially-manufactured toilet paper doubled in duty to carry the written word. The Friends Library in Euston, England has a magazine written entirely on prison toilet paper by pacifist prisoners, whose literary activities resulted in prison reform. Some countries' toilet papers, such as Czechoslovakia's, resemble writing paper, and are used as such by amused tourists. Germany's Starlite Tissue Company produced toilet paper with English language lessons on it.

The widespread use of toilet paper has created a problem for governments and public service-providers: pilferage. Mexico has adopted the most straightforward solution; their airports and bus stations simply don't provide any paper, and unprepared travelers soon learn to carry their own. Scandinavian countries have a partial solution; their rolls are too big to conceal, so any stealing has to be on a handful-by-handful basis. H. M. Stationery Office of the British Government and the German rail system imprint institution names on each sheet they provide, presumably to shame would-be thieves into, at the very least, not providing stolen paper to house-guests, utilizing the same principle hotels use in personalizing their towels.

The international variety in toilet paper is no less impressive than the range of theft-deterring techniques. The U.S. has the softest and most absorbent, in white, pastels, or prints, sometimes even embossed with little flowers and scented. German paper is often light gray. Some European papers have a rough side as well as a glazed, shiny side with which to apply the final polish.

But even specialized toilet paper isn't the end-

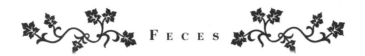

point in the evolution of our tools. The march of technology has inspired many to seek alternatives to dry paper. In Europe, many upscale citizens have started to carry and use special foil-wrapped moist wipes like the disposable moist towelettes that come with airplane meals and boxes of fried chicken. Meanwhile, pharmaceutical companies are currently working on a diet-aid that inhibits the metabolization of fats, and one of its side effects is greasier, smellier stools. If the drug ever comes to market, the popularity of these foil-wrapped moist towelettes will undoubtedly increase.

Toilet fixtures are also evolving to readdress the perineal cleansing issue. American Standard manufactures a toilet based on Alexander Kira's ergonomic and forest-friendly modified squat-plates with buttock support and bidet-like cleansing water jet. The most high-tech designs come from Japan, however. There, over 12% of homes now have ultra-sophisticated new toilets with built-in hot-water cleansing and hot-air drying mechanisms, and the percentage increases each year. Some prototypes even have diagnostic equipment and telecommunication ports to link to hospital computers.

Meanwhile, the murder of our forests for TP and other paper products has prompted many people to support cultivation of kenaf and hemp, both of which produce far more paper-per-acre than trees. Another simpler approach is just to use less; three squares per wad is plenty! During the dock strike in Hawaii in 1973, which caused numerous shortages, authorities recommended using no more than three squares. Navy TP dispensers in Hawaii also allow only three squares at a time (although there's usually one roll with the peg filed down or ripped out to allow a freer flow).

Some timber-conscious Oregon residents are taking the most ambitious approach of all by promoting the idea of phasing out toilet paper entirely, substituting thimbleberry leaves or, as suggested in the newsletter of the Aprovecho Institute of Cottage Grove, Oregon, the age-old hand-and-water method. You always go back to the basics.

Constipation: An American Obsession

Corn flakes and graham crackers: food just doesn't get more All-American than these two crunchy favorites. Unlike hot dogs and pizza, corn flakes and graham crackers were invented right here in the U.S. by two men, John Harvey Kellogg and Sylvester Graham, who alike drew their culinary inspiration from a common, also characteristically American obsession: regularity of stool. Both of these manufactured grain-products come from and hearken back to a unique era in the development of our national psyche, an Anal Age, roughly 1870-1935, during which concern about changing life-styles, interest in self-improvement, sexual repression, and plain old Puritan fanaticism/kookiness focused much of the public's attention on the perfectionist task of ensuring prompt and regular defecation at all times. People before and since, especially since, have likewise been interested in regularity, but it was during this Anal Age, in this country, that the concern reached its zenith, and the obsession with regularity that people from other countries still find so amusing in us owes much to Kellogg, Graham, and the many other visionaries of this unique age.

Two historical trains of influence collided during the Anal Age. The first one, belief in the healing power of enemas, may have originated with the Essenes, a health-conscious religious sect active in Palestine during Roman times. A 3rd Century A.D. Aramaic document, *The Essene Gospel of Peace*, warns, "I tell you truly, the uncleanness within is greater by much than the uncleanness without." To combat this evil, it recommends that you find a gourd with a trailing stalk, hollow it out, fill it with warm water, "suffer the end of the stalk of the trailing gourd to enter your hinder parts, that the water may flow through all your bowels," and then, finally, "let the water run out from your body, that it may carry away from within it all the unclean and evil-smelling things of Satan."

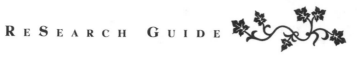

The enema train continued on to Germany in the 15th Century, when an influential doctor named Johann Kämpf hopped aboard. Kämpf first propounded the "doctrine of the infarctus," which held that fecal impaction was the cause of most human diseases. Dr. Kämpf's cure for most diseases, logically, was enemas, or "clysters." Many doctors subscribed to this new doctrine, and in addition also held that the body could absorb nutrients from enemas, adding further to their perceived health benefits.

Economic progress powered the second train. We know that "richer" foods, highly refined foods heavy on fat and low on roughage, are more likely to cause constipation. During prehistoric times, our instinct to seek fat in our diet helped us survive, because the only foods available were unrefined foods, and by following our cravings we usually wound up with a reasonably healthy diet. However, the same fat-seeking instincts began serving people less well once they learned how to refine foods to taste, removing roughage and boosting the fat levels.

But very few people could eat these refined foods. As the adjective suggests, "rich" foods, were only available to the wealthy. In the 1600's, probably as the result of the rich diet as well as the usual idleness and self-absorption, clysters made from a variety of recipes became all the rage among the nobility in Europe. Even after the mid-1800's, by which time scientists had determined that the body derived no nourishment from enemas, they remained as popular as ever. If Freud's Wolf Man is an indication, by the turn of the century, a number of troubled aristocrats had come to depend on enemas psychologically, even to the point of addiction, quite apart from perceiving that they had any health benefits.

But economic development changed the situation. As the society increased its wealth and raised its overall standard of living, a richer diet resembling the one formerly enjoyed only by the aristocracy became available to more people. And as the eating habits of the rich became available to the middle class, so did some of its other habits. This is where the two trains met. Suddenly, large numbers of people had a constipating diet and were looking at enemas, and more drastic measures, as the solution.

Dr. Sylvester Graham (1794-1851) was a man ahead of his time. He took up the Kämpf doctrine in this country and laid much of the groundwork that Kellogg and others would later build upon. Graham was zealous about keeping the bowels moving swiftly, and maintained that this precaution would ensure health, largely through the prevention of masturbation. It is to this man's imagination that we owe the development of graham flour (derived from whole wheat flour), used to make graham crackers.

In 1870, a Dr. W. W. Hall published an early book typical of the era, *Health and Disease, As Affected By Constipation and its Unmedicinal Cure*. Dr. Hall wrote that ideally, people should defecate once per day, after breakfast, and at the same time each day. "Nor should persons sit long at stool," he explains, "Less than ten minutes should include the whole operation." Loose bowels, he felt, are best treated with opium!

As the Anal Age progressed, health-obsessed Americans focused increasingly more energy on prompt defecation, relying on enemas, medicines, and even surgery. Changing diet and prosperity were factors propelling people toward this concern, but other forces drove it much further: aggressive advertising by laxative manufacturers, practice-building by doctors and others who made a living administering weekly enemas to the fashionable, and fanatical demagogues who somehow touched a nerve when they preached that all but the busiest of bathroom-visitation schedules spelled life-threatening constipation. Fed by these influences, bowel regularity became an obsession for the era's hypochondriac neurotics, and a source of concern for more normal people, much as diet and exercise are today.

In 1917, Dr. John H. Kellogg and the Good Health Publishing Company of Battle Creek, Michigan, published another typical Anal Age work, *Colon Hygiene*. Kellogg, the superintendent of the large sanitarium in Battle Creek, had written about health matters before; his astonishingly monotonous *Plain Facts For Old and Young*, a family guide he wrote back in 1881 with a zeal characteristic of tightly-channeled, youthful energies, devotes nearly half of its 428 pages to the evils and ruinous dangers of masturbation, sandwiching warning upon warning between terrifying case histories and rounds of scathing invective against all practitioners of The Solitary Vice. His thesis in *Colon Hygiene*, however, shared by his other books *Auto-Intoxication or Intestinal Toxemia* and *The Itinerary of a Breakfast*, covers different territory. It starts out reasonably enough; Kellogg states that the "civilized" diet of meats, sauces, and a few cooked vegetables does not match the length of our colons, which are better suited to rougher fare. But Kellogg goes on to assert that as a result, a toxic putrefaction of wastes takes place in our descending colon, poisoning our blood and, consequently, our entire bodies. This poisoning occurs during constipation, which Kellogg calls the "most common and most destructive disease of civilized peoples."

Constipation can—nay, must—be cured, according to Kellogg, by proper sleep habits, baths, enemas, good posture, surgery (a colon "short-circuiting" operation, about which more later), and of course diet, and with this last point, Kellogg made his greatest contribution to our culture. The doctor recommended a diet of milk and half-cooked grains or bran, and this led him to develop Corn Flakes and other cereals. His brother went into business manufacturing these toasted grain-adjuncts to milk, giving birth to the now-enormous Kellogg Company, which still operates out of Battle Creek.

In *Colon Hygiene*, Kellogg gives dietary recommendations, exercises, and recipes for various enemas, including hot water, hot soap, saline, sugar water, paraffin oil, alum, and glycerin, but above all he emphasizes the importance of timely defecation. With a religious fervor he writes, "The prompt evacuation of the bowels in response to Nature's 'call' is a sacred obligation which no person can neglect without serious injury." He concludes the book with his 18-point "Colon Code," the first two commandments of which are, "Move the bowels at least three times a day," and, "Answer the 'call,' even the slightest, at once. Delay of five or ten minutes may be disastrous."

Kellogg had a number of like-minded contemporaries, including Dr. W. H. Graves and Sir Arbuthnot Lane. In 1930, Dr. Graves claimed that 90% of all illnesses stemmed from constipation, and held that proper defecation was more necessary for good health than proper eating. Americans, Graves felt, should stop asking, "When do we eat?" and start asking, "How well do we eliminate?" Sir Arbuthnot Lane, meanwhile, pioneered the surgical removal of a large part of the colon, thus making it better-suited to the modern diet. Several other doctors followed his lead, and Kellogg himself recommended and performed the procedure, about which he wrote, "Of the 22,000 operations I have personally performed, I have never found a single normal colon." To the public's credit, however, the procedure never caught on widely.

In the 1920's, enemas achieved fad status. Serious devotees could opt for a newly popular procedure: high colonic irrigation, which filled the entire colon with water, instead of merely the rectum. Many wealthy partisans visited doctors regularly to receive their irrigations, and at least one of these practitioners is reported to have kept a set of flasks handy in his office, each of which contained some noxious-looking mass which he would exhibit to his patients afterwards, with the claim that he had just washed it out of their systems.

Swept up with the mood of the times, scientists started experimenting with enemas. In 1932, in a sort of backdoor-Pavlovian study, French scientists demonstrated that after giving cats 20 to 28 enemas while sounding a particular note, the sounding of the note alone would induce the felines to defecate.

Meanwhile, the laxative industry capitalized on this obsession with proper elimination. During the Great Depression, when radio couldn't afford to be too picky about its sponsors, it started to accept more laxative commercials. The ads succeeded brilliantly; one campaign, "Madam X, the

Ex-Lax Reporter," was estimated to have sold 40 million boxes of Ex-Lax in a single year. Programs of dance music carried commercial interruptions with tag lines like, "If Nature forgets, remember Ex-Lax." Other companies joined in to peddle such remedies as Fletcher's Castoria and Crazy Water Crystals, and even Fleischmann's got into the game. One commercial ended with the whisper of a young woman sitting with her beau in the moonlight: "Darling, if you're constipated, take Fleischmann's Yeast."

Many listeners telephoned the radio companies to complain about these spots, some of which discussed bodily symptoms in unflinching detail. In response, in 1935, CBS president William S. Paley prohibited his stations from broadcasting laxative ads or any other "socially unacceptable" material. Ex-Lax was not pleased with the new policy, but it (and all other laxative companies) responded by simply moving their sponsorship over to NBC, which soon became the network known for having all the laxative ads.

Today, medical consensus tells us that defecating between three times a day and once every three days is within the range of healthy normalcy, and while few can deny the unpleasantness of constipation, we don't hear voices telling us it's fatal anymore. Ironically, actual dangers: hernia, prolapse of the rectum, and even stroke, result from hurriedly straining to push out refractory stools (Valsalva's maneuver) rather than relaxing. Nevertheless, echoes of the Anal Age are still with us. Alexander Kira, calling constipation "The Great American Disease," cites a survey showing that two-thirds of the American public believe a daily stool is necessary and one-third believe it prudent to do something regularly to ensure a daily stool. Nutritionists, herbalists, holistic healers, and others recommend a wide range of enemas and high colonics, and television commercials for Ex-Lax and Metamucil fill the air. In 1976 a man named Ernest Whitford ran for President on the platform that the country needed more bran in its diet, because ending constipation, the number one cause of stress, would reduce disease and crime.

Most of us would probably prefer not to "miss a day," but ironically, the solution might be to relax, stop worrying about the problem, and quit taking laxatives and enemas. Many professionals and business executives today, who wolf down junk food and can't relax for a few minutes on the toilet, suffer from constipation, or what recent medical literature, typifying baby-boom self-importance and disconnectedness, has renamed "Young Executive Tight Sphincter Syndrome." One expert, Dr. Stephen Wexner, advises his YETSS patients to simply eat more roughage, drink more liquids, and avoid habitually taking laxatives or enemas, which the colon can come to depend on like addictive agents. An enema or laxative abuser who doesn't get a "fix" may be constipated for a week, and this can lead to a cycle of dependence that's difficult to break. But as with any other addictive agents, laxatives and enemas may tend to attract obsessive, fringe-element, eccentric genius types who, despite (or maybe because of) their chemical dependencies make lasting creative contributions to society. Also, it has been suggested that colonics can be unhealthy; if the equipment is not perfectly sterile, toxins may be spread, resulting in a fatality. Ponder this over your next bowl of breakfast cereal.

Coprolites

Ordinarily, feces decomposes and returns to the earth to nourish another generation of life, but the occasional stool sidesteps this eternal cycle and remains preserved long after its maker, and perhaps even its maker's civilization, has died. Not surprisingly, these fossilized turds, coprolites, can provide anthropologists with detailed information about what prehistoric people ate and how they lived.

The best, most highly-prized coprolites come from caves, shelters, or tombs where they've dried out and remained undisturbed. As early as 1910, scientists began breaking apart and examining specimens of fossilized feces found in mummies and caves. But this crude technique was just the beginning.

In 1955, "dry analysis" gave way to rehydration, in which the stool is soaked in an aqueous solution of trisodium phosphate (TSP, a common cleanser) for a few days, and then sliced, separated, centrifuged, sniffed, screened through series of sieves, stained and smeared on slides, sent to the lab, and otherwise studied to reveal food remains, chemical composition, pollen, parasites, particles, and other telling traits. As an added advantage, rehydration can reveal whether the stool is of human origin. Human scats turn the immersion fluid a characteristic opaque, dark brown or black. The only other animal whose dried dung produces this distinctive color is the Coatimundi, also an omnivore. Without this test, you only know a coprolite is human if it came from a tomb or contains identifiable eggs or bodies of exclusively human parasites, such as *Enterobius vermicularis* or *Ascaris lumbricoides*.

One leading paleo-scatologist, Dr. Andrew Jones of England's University of York, has taken the field even further by varying his diet until his own stools match the ones he studies. As part of his Ph.D. work, he ate kippers and studied the digested bones. Later, he went on a high-fiber diet to see how closely he could counterfeit the feces left by the Vikings—except for the parasites.

Naturally, scats reveal what foods people ate. Fibrous vegetable matter identifies itself easily. Meat is more difficult to detect, but bone particles give it away. Some interesting foods found through coprolite analysis include insects, bone meal cooked in fat, and herbivore browse (semi-digested plant matter taken from the stomach of an herbivorous animal).

Coprolites can also reveal how the foods were prepared. Grit indicates milling. Charcoal indicates parching or roasting. Meanwhile, parasites shed light on habits and living conditions. There can be informative surprises as well, such as the coprolite found in Danger Cave, Utah, which consisted almost entirely of the bark of the red osier dogwood, which was used as a narcotic.

If the feces is excavated from latrines, anthro-pologists learn even more. People have always used commodes to dispose of more than just human waste, so these sites often carry a variety of well-preserved artifacts which paint a particularly honest picture of the lives that left them behind, because their discarders never intended for them to be found.

Enough people know this, and participate in such excavations themselves, to support an organization called the National Privy Diggers Association. One amateur privy-digger has unearthed Model-T parts, ice skates, bicycles, billiard balls and false teeth, as well as the usual array of intact and broken glassware and china.

The real finds, however, are the very old coprolites themselves. For example, the Archaeological Resource Center in York, England, displays what may be the most valuable piece of shit in the world: the Lloyds Bank Turd. Discovered under a Lloyds Bank building and subsequently assessed at a value of £20,000, the Turd is an almost mint-condition, 1000-year-old human stool. Freud would have loved it.

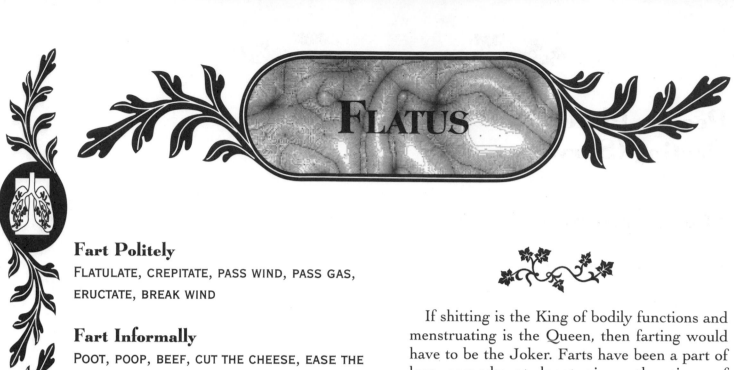

FLATUS

Fart Politely

FLATULATE, CREPITATE, PASS WIND, PASS GAS, ERUCTATE, BREAK WIND

Fart Informally

POOT, POOP, BEEF, CUT THE CHEESE, EASE THE BREEZE, KWATZ, BLOW, LIFT A LEG, MAKE A SMELLY, RIP/CUT ONE, TALK GERMAN (OLD BRITISH SLANG)

A Fart

SPIDER BARK, ROUSER, SILENT BUT DEADLY (S.B.D.), CARPET CREEPER

A Fart Noise

BRONX CHEER, RASPBERRY

If shitting is the King of bodily functions and menstruating is the Queen, then farting would have to be the Joker. Farts have been a part of low comedy at least since the time of Aristophanes, and one of the greatest farters of all time, Joseph Pujol, wisely employed his unique talent as a performer. Pujol's windy anal antics routinely had turn-of-the-century audiences rolling in the aisles.

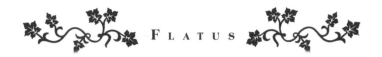

People, Places, and Pooting (Survey)

Flatus Expulsion Section

About how many times per day do you usually fart?

The widest gender gap in the entire survey divides the answers to this question. The average reported daily fart quotient is 9.15, but women's estimates average 3.28 per day while the men's average 13.63. In addition, twelve men and only one woman (12% of sample) answer nonquantitatively along the lines of "plenty," "a lot," "many," etc.

Longer comments also reflect the estimated fart rate gender gap. A young man writes, "A better question might be how many times am I not farting." Another answers, "Seems practically constant, I think I'm abnormal." One more estimates "Once every ten minutes," a guess which, allowing for eight uncounted hours of sleep, translates to 96 farts/day, the highest rate in the sample. Second place is occupied by two more men, who give 35 and 30-40 as averages.

Meanwhile, a 20-year-old woman who estimates that she farts at least four times per day, a lower bound for most men, explains that this "high" frequency stems from her high fiber diet. Women dominate the low end of the range, with three of them answering that on most days they don't fart at all and one more estimating her average fart rate at twice weekly.

What foods do you associate with flatulence (besides the obvious ones)?

Despite the question's obviousness exemption, beans, bean soups, and "canned bean products" garner the most votes here, with 17%. Next in rankness rank beer, with 9%, and then coffee and onions, with 8% each. 8% total also mention dairy products, as a class or in ice cream, yogurt, milk, and cheese specifically. Another 8% answer

"none" or say they have no food-fart associations.

Ingestibles getting 5% of the vote or less include, in descending order of mention, cabbage and sauerkraut, garlic, apples, legumes and seeds other than beans (peanuts, chickpeas, lentils, and raw sunflower seeds), Mexican food, meat, dried foods, chocolate, bananas, colas, LSD, greasy pizza, salad, eggs, "Natural-type foods," tropical fruit, fast food, chicken, oatmeal cookies, oat bran, fish, spaghetti, hot dogs, Slim Fast, broccoli, Grape Nuts cereal, the "25¢ Meal" (a salad, spaghetti, soup and bread meal served for a quarter by a Bushspeak "point of light" in Berkeley, California), and, finally, "Any radical change in diet, like from dorm food to home cooked." One 20-year-old self-described "drug advocate" observes that, "Beer and LSD give you those 'smoothies' that go quietly but cause trouble."

In what social situations do you allow yourself to fart? In situations in which you hold it back, when do you finally let it go (bathroom visit, outside, end of evening, crowded dance floor . . .)? Do you generally excuse yourself or otherwise say anything to acknowledge it? What do you say?

About equal numbers of respondents say they do and do not avoid farting in social situations. Some of those who do not say they have little choice in the matter. Explains one young architecture student, "Doesn't seem like farts can be held off until later — I'll excuse myself and go pinch a loaf if it's really ridiculous." A young woman who reports farting three to four times per day writes, "I can't hold mine back usually ever. I often tell people I've farted."

Survey participants discuss a variety of do- and don't-fart situations and settings. They confirm the list parenthesized in the question (bathroom visit, etc.) and add, in decreasing order of mention: with friends and mates, when no one is near, when no one will notice, with same-sex friends, while walking, riding a bicycle, or otherwise "in motion," around family or relatives, where there's good ventilation, when it's noisy, at campfires or barbecues (a "must" according to one teen), at

parties, and after having left the room for a moment. A male grad student writes, "If only my male friends are present, I make a pre-fart announcement to get their attention, and then go for volume." A geologist explains that he farts around "old girlfriends—never new ones, old friends, certain relatives, [and] nuns."

Places and situations in which people don't fart are: all social situations, on dates, during sex, at dinner with parents' friends, in bed, with new girl- or boyfriends, and in conference with the boss. Explains one 22-year-old man, "Worst situation is sleeping (not fucking, sleeping) with a new girlfriend. By morning, there is usually major buildup."

12% of respondents say they sometimes intentionally make their farts silent to maintain anonymity, and 2% say they sometimes cover up the noise with coughs or other mouth sounds. A 26-year-old boasts, "I'm extremely good at letting farts out quietly." A more cautious young man writes, "I'm pretty sneaky, or so I think." A 24-year-old fellow explains, "I do my best to disguise it. This requires some prognostication. If I feel it's gonna 'rumble,' I try to create a sound of equal dissonance (throat clearing, other stertorous noises). If I feel a 'buzz,' I'll fake a sneeze. If I guess incorrectly, I'm fucked."

9% report that they'll say "excuse me," particularly if they think their fart has not escaped notice. Other respondents list different apologies, acknowledgments, and warnings, including "Whoops!," "Yow!," "Sorry," "Open a window," "Watch out for the aftershocks," and "Whee! Is there a stain on my trousers?" A grad student studying acoustic perception remarks that he and his girlfriend "often comment on any outstanding attributes (flavor, pungency, etc. and amplitude, duration or modulation of the sound)." A polite woman writes that she announces "Courtesy Walk" beforehand. Meanwhile, a 27-year-old takes a dim view of those who own up, writing, "People who call attention to themselves are the type who fought for gold stars in grammar school."

A teenage boy explains that he will, if detected,

"acknowledge that the dog did it." In all, 4% of responses mention blaming others or acting as if someone else did it.

Two confident young women write that others never smell or otherwise notice their farts. Two young men, meanwhile, explain that their social farting decisions depend on, as one of them puts it, "how pungent the current crop is. If they're real powerful, I'll hold 'em in." Finally, an Englishman jokes, "The answer to this is far more long-winded than I have time for."

(Singles:) How long (if at all) do you have to be "going out" with someone before you'll fart in their company? Or do you just wait for them to go first? How long do they typically take? (Marrieds:) Do you fart freely in the presence of your spouse when there's just the two of you there?

Many respondents who classify themselves as single for this question answer in general terms like "a while" and "it varies," but thirty give specific times, ranging from no time to one year. The average wait time comes out to 92.77 days, 62.98 days for the men and 149.82 days for the women. Others answer in terms of number of dates, ranging from one to twenty.

11% say they won't or try not to fart at all (including: "I can't beef with cute chicks around—I need help!" and "Haven't ever farted comfortably or admittedly with a guy in my presence.") 6% write that when they begin farting depends on the person or the relationship (including: "It's not time, but depth of knowledge," and "After we've slept together and I like and trust them."). Meanwhile, 6% simply answer that they don't know how long they typically take.

Three young women answer that it doesn't matter how long they take because their companions never notice it anyway.

8% say they don't wait for the other party, while 1% say they do. As for how long the romantic interest in question takes, most who answer say they don't know or that it varies.

Of those who answer as "Marrieds" (many of whom are legally single but live with mates), twelve of fifteen say they do fart freely around their honeys, and some even do it for fun. One woman explains, "We *try* to fart—free entertainment!" Similarly, a middle-aged man writes that sometimes he and his wife "engage in farting/belching contests." On the other side, a woman of 29 answers, "No, I would rather go to the bathroom if I have the time," and a 41-year-old man answers, "No, but my wife does."

Ever ignite a fart? What color did it glow? Did you singe any hairs?

Only 12% of respondents, all men, report having done this. 2% say they've only witnessed the activity. Colors observed, in descending frequency order, are blue/bluish, blue-orange, orange, red-orange, and green-orange. Three say they singed hairs, four say they did not, and two don't know, one of them explaining, "It wasn't my butt."

A 31-year-old student writes, "Have a friend who got second degree burns up there." A 28-year-old relates that her father and his college buddies, "once got drunk and started lighting their farts. The flame went right up one guy's butt and he jumped out the window and broke his leg!" A baker/student/fine artist of 31 answers, "No, but my mom's brother did—it ignited T.P. in bowl and it cracked the toilet lid (the fire)!" Finally, a machinist/engineer/wizard of 47 recalls, "I saw a guy in the Army do himself some pretty serious defuzzing like that . . . . Shot flame about two feet out his ass."

It's clear from people's comments that the "safe" way to light farts is to leave your trousers on.

Ever fart onto your hand? Did you sniff your hand afterwards? Were you at all surprised? Do you think this is sick behavior?

21% say they have farted into their hands. 15% say they sniffed their hands afterwards. Only 3% say it surprised them, and 10% say they consider the behavior "sick."

Most comments address the "sickness" issue. Some consider the behavior downright healthy, like the 26-year-old who answers, "Not at all. Curiosity is a healthy trait." Others offer differ-

ent terms: distasteful, boorish, twisted, weird, and a bit odd. A 23-year-old gives the opinion that it's not sick unless it's habitual. Finally, a wise 20-year-old woman asks, "Why analyze it?"

Explanations and related experiences participants share include, "My brother once farted in the bathtub and caught the fart in a glass jar," and, "Jean Genet writes about this in *Our Lady of the Flowers*."

Ever fart while swimming? Were you wearing a skin-tight bathing suit? A wetsuit? Did anyone comment, or did they just pretend not to notice?

71% say they have, having done it in tight and baggy swimsuits, wetsuits, and nude. A 30-year-old adds that he "once pissed in a wetsuit," and a 24-year-old remarks, "I've taken a shit in a lake, if that means anything."

Most of the time, it seems, others don't seem to notice or at least don't comment, but two respondents recall that when they were on swim teams, team members made a game of farting. Several people report what one young man describes as a "nice effervescent feeling."

Finally, a knowledgeable 32-year-old student asks, "Ever hear of 'gut squeeze'? It's supposedly a malady some people get scuba diving after eating gas-producing foods; after being at depth for a while and ascending, the gas in your gut expands rapidly, causing much farting and distress."

Ever "blame" someone else for one of your farts? Ever been in a situation in which everyone comments, but no one admits responsibility? Was it in a car?

52% say they have blamed others, suggesting that what may be one of humankind's oldest lies is also one of its most widespread. Some even say they blame others as policy. Respondents single out siblings, children, dogs, and cats as prime targets.

One man writes, "I have a habit of pointing accusingly at people on the bus." A 30-year-old archaeologist informs, "There's an expression in Spanish: 'He's so unscrupulous that if he farted

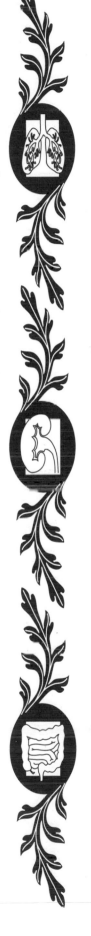

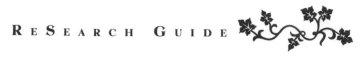

at a wake, he'd blame it on the cadaver.'" An older man recounts a true story not too dissimilar: "Once when a youngster at a church, I had a really big fart, and figured that I could just lean over a little bit and slide it out quietly. Of course, it wouldn't cooperate-operate . . . . There was this tremendous BRAAAACK!, and thinking *very* quickly I turned around and looked at the kid behind me. It was *very* difficult not to blow my cover by giggling."

67% say they've been in the no-one-admits-it situation. Most of them say it happened in a car, but respondents also mention camp, the subway, in a tent, in a small room, in an elementary school classroom, while watching television, at parties, in a cafeteria, and, from a 27-year-old lawyer, in hotel rooms. Meanwhile, a 20-year-old woman answers, "No. I hang with honest folks."

Finally, the man who farted loudly as a youngster in church tells another story: "In the early 60's I was a dragster. It became great sport to see who could force the rest of the folks in the tow-car into opening the windows first while traveling to/from races. We'd stop and tank up with chili, corned beef and cabbage, hard-boiled eggs, and draft beer for more fuel for the fart-wars. I'm surprised that the upholstery survived."

Joseph Pujol, the Fartiste

One summer's day in the mid-1860's, a young French boy named Joseph Pujol had a frightening experience at the seashore. Swimming out alone, he held his breath and dove underwater. Suddenly an icy cold feeling penetrated his gut. Frightened, he ran ashore, but then received a second shock when he noticed seawater streaming from his anus. The experience so disturbed the lad that his mother took him to a doctor to allay his fears. The doctor complied.

The boy didn't know it at the time, but this unsettling rectal experience at the beach not only indicated no illness, but it also foretold of a gift that would later make him the toast of Paris and one of the most popular and successful performers of his generation.

Joseph Pujol was born in Marseilles on June 1, 1857 to Francois Pujol and Rose Demaury, a respected stonemason/sculptor and his wife, both of whom had emigrated from Catalan. Young Joseph went to school until the age of 13, whereupon he apprenticed himself to a baker. Several years later, he served in the French army.

While in the army, he mentioned his childhood sea-bathing experience to his buddies. They immediately wanted to know if he could do it again, so on a day's leave soon afterward he went out to the shore to swim and experiment. He successfully reenacted the hydraulics of his childhood experience there and even discovered that by contracting his abdomen muscles, he could intentionally take up as much water as he liked and eject it in a powerful stream. Demonstrating this ability back at the barracks later provided the soldiers with no end of amusement, and soon Pujol started to practice with air instead of water, giving him the ability to produce a variety of sounds. This new development provided even more enjoyment for his buddies. It was then and there, in the army, that Pujol invented a nickname for himself that would later become a stage name synonymous throughout Europe with helpless, hysterical laughter: "Le Petomane" (translation: "The Fartiste").

After his stint in the army, Pujol returned to Marseilles and to a bakery his father set him up in, on a street that, today, proudly bears the name "rue Pujol." At the age of 26 he married Elizabeth Henriette Oliver, the 20-year-old daughter of a local butcher. Pujol enjoyed performing, so in the evenings he entertained at local music halls by singing, doing comedy routines, and even playing his trombone backstage between numbers. He continued amusing his friends privately with his "other" wind instrument, but only at their suggestion and urging did he decide to turn this parlor trick into a full-fledged act for public audiences.

Pujol worked up a Le Petomane routine, and with some friends he rented a space in Marseilles to perform it in. They promoted the show heavily themselves through posters and handouts, but word-of-mouth soon took over and they packed the house every night. *Fin de siècle* European audiences, deeply repressed but newly prosperous and trying to be "modern"—the same people Freud observed (Freud was one year older than Pujol)—must have found a man on stage building an entire act out of mock farting and other forms of anal play considerably more shockingly funny than we would today. Pujol's was a good act by any era's standards, but back then his scatology hit especially hard. Like Alfred Jarry, whose momentous, scatological *Ubu Roi* actually post-dates Pujol's Paris debut by several years, Pujol was a French Revolutionary of the modern theater. Jarry gets the credit today because he was a "serious playwright" and not a lowbrow cabaret performer, but Pujol clearly laid some of the groundwork.

Word-of-mouth spread reports of the quality and uniqueness of Pujol's new show, and soon people from all over Marseilles were coming to see it.

After the hometown success, Pujol's friends urged him to take the act to Paris. Pujol hoped to, but cautiously decided to play several other provincial cities first to refine the act and test the breadth of its appeal before taking it to the capital. He performed in Toulon, Bordeaux, and Clermont-Ferrand with great success, and in 1892 was finally ready to try his act at Paris's Moulin Rouge. It was then that Pujol reputedly uttered a line oft-repeated in cabaret lore; looking up at the windmill sails of the landmark Moulin Rouge ("Red Mill") building, he exclaimed, "The sails of the Moulin Rouge—what a marvelous fan for my act!"

In getting booked at the Moulin Rouge, Pujol wasted no time. He walked in and demanded to see the director with such confidence that the secretary showed him in immediately. He then told the director, a man named either Zidler or Oller depending on whose account you follow (I'll use "Oller"), "I am Le Petomane, and I want an engagement in your establishment." He said that

he was a phenomenon and that his gift would be the talk of Paris. When Oller asked for an explanation, he calmly replied, "You see, sir, my anus is of such elasticity that I can open and shut it at will . . . . I can absorb any quantity of liquid I may be given . . . [and] I can expel an almost infinite quantity of odorless gas." After this, he gave Oller a quick demonstration.

Oller put Pujol on stage that very night.

Pujol dressed formally for his act, wearing a coat, red breeches, white stockings, gloves, and patent leather shoes—a stuffy, old-fashioned outfit that , coupled with his unrelenting, deadpan delivery, must have lent an abrasive comedic dissonance to the actual content of his performance. To begin his act he introduced himself and explained that he was about to demonstrate the art of "petomanie." He further explained that he could break wind at will, but assured his audience not to worry because his parents had "ruined themselves" in scenting his rectum.

Le Petomane used the simple, honest format of announcing and then demonstrating some imitations. He displayed his wide sonic range with tenor, baritone, and bass fart sounds. He imitated the farts of a little girl, a mother-in-law, a bride on her wedding night (tiny), the same bride the day after (loud), and a mason (dry—"no cement"). He imitated thunder, cannons ("Gunners stand by your guns! Ready—fire!"), and even the sound of a dressmaker tearing two yards of calico (a full 10-second rip). After the imitations, Le Petomane popped backstage to put one end of a yard-long rubber tube into his anus. He returned and smoked a cigarette from this tube, after which he used it to play a couple of tunes on a song flute. For his finale he removed the rubber tube, blew out some of the gas-jet footlights from a safe distance away, and then led the audience in a rousing sing-along.

This first night, a few tightly-corseted women in the audience literally fainted from laughing so hard. Oller immediately gave Pujol a contract to perform at the Moulin Rouge, elsewhere in France, and abroad. Turning audience-fainting into a great gimmick, Oller later conspicuously

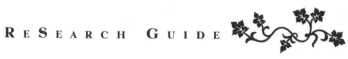

stationed white-uniformed nurses in the hall at each Le Petomane show and instructed them to carry out any audience members rendered particularly helpless by the hilarity. Meanwhile, to quash any rumors that his performance was faked, Pujol occasionally gave private men-only performances clad in a bathing suit with a large hole in the seat rather than his concealing regular costume.

It was after one of these private performances that a distinguished-looking man put a 20 franc gold coin in the collection plate. When Pujol questioned him, he turned out to be the King of Belgium, who had come incognito just to see his act.

After signing up with the Moulin Rouge in 1892, Pujol moved his growing family (starting in 1885, Pujol and his wife had a child every two years for eighteen years) into a chalet staffed by servants who soon became family friends. As he predicted, he became the talk of Paris, and admirers saluted him affectionately as he rode by in his carriage. Paris doctors examined him and published an article in *La Semaine Médicale* that described his health but offered no new explanation for his ability. It did however record that he could rectally project a jet of water 4 to 5 yards. Box office receipts alone attest to Le Petomane's popularity. One Sunday the Moulin Rouge took in 20,000 francs for a Le Petomane performance, an amount which dwarfs the 8000 francs typically grossed by Sarah Bernhardt at the peak of her career there.

But another thing happened in 1892 that provoked a series of battles between Pujol and Moulin Rouge management, the litigious nature of which makes it sound more like 1992. Pujol visited a friend of his who sold gingerbread, and to attract customers to his friend's stall, he did some Petomane tricks right there in the marketplace. Word of this "unauthorized performance" got back to Oller, who took it up with Pujol and threatened to sue. Over the next couple of years, Pujol, who dreamed of opening up his own traveling theater, had more rows with Oller. In 1894, Oller brought suit against Pujol over the gingerbread stall incident and won. Pujol was fined 3000

Francs. The next year, Pujol left the Moulin Rouge to start his own venture, the Theatre Pompadour. Soon after Pujol left, the Moulin Rouge put up a new act, billed as a "Woman Petomane" (they concealed a bellows under her skirt). Pujol then brought a lawsuit against the Moulin Rouge for plagiarizing his idea. At about the same time, however, a newspaper panned the "Woman Petomane" act, and the actress, Angele Thiebeau, sued the paper for libel. The judgment against Thiebeau was so harshly worded and humiliating that Pujol, satisfied at the harm done to the Moulin Rouge's reputation, withdrew his own lawsuit against them.

Pujol's new Theatre Pompadour included mime and magic and other acts performed by Pujol's family and performer friends. He changed his own act into a woodland tale told in doggerel punctuated at the end of each couplet by Le Petomane sound effects and imitations of the animal and bird characters in the story. Paris audiences liked the winning charm of this home-grown variety show and still yucked it up at Pujol's fart noises, so the Theater Pompadour prospered for many years.

Le Petomane continued to be an enormous draw in his new venue until around 1900, when the interest of the show-going public began to wane. The Pompadour continued to do pretty well, however, until World War I, when four of Pujol's sons went off to fight and the theater had to close down. One son was taken prisoner and two of the others became invalids, and Pujol was so shattered that after the war he had no interest in returning to his performing career. The family moved back to Marseilles and Pujol ran bakeries with his sons and unmarried daughters. In 1922, he and his family moved to Toulon and he set up a biscuit factory which he gave to his children to manage. He lived the rest of his life there, surrounded by his many dearly loved children and grandchildren. His wife died in 1930 and he died in 1945. One medical school offered the family 25,000 francs to be allowed to examine his body, but out of respect, reverence and love for this warm, funny, and caring man, not one of his children agreed to let them.

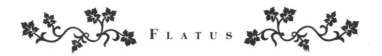

On Farting

Nitrogen, oxygen, and carbon dioxide provide the vehicle. Hydrogen and methane make it flame. Its primary identity comes from hydrogen sulfide (the "rotten egg" gas), while small amounts of more complex chemicals such as indole and skatole give it individual personality. That's what it is. That's all it is. Yet, like snowflakes, each fart is a little bit different.

The nitrogen and oxygen, the two least interesting components, come from swallowed air, and if you eat too quickly, sigh a lot, breathe abnormally, or chew gum, you may be adding to the bulk of your blasts without increasing their potency.

Because the more complex, volatile chemicals that give farts their character are produced by intestinal bacteria as they break down various proteins, complex sugars, and fats, it's the foods you eat that largely determine what your farts will be like. Which foods have the greatest effect on your wind depends on your own individual nature, but some common ones are broccoli, onions, cauliflower, cabbage, radishes, apples, candy, fried foods, nuts, raisins, berries, carbonated beverages (for volume only), spices, licorice, alcohol, tomatoes, beans, milk, cheese, bran, cucumbers, coffee, eggs, Brussels sprouts, and beer, particularly dark beer.

According to a quaint and questionable experiment done during the fart's scientific research heyday, the late 1700's, the air that surrounds you also affects the character of your farts, and not just because they contain swallowed air. Describing the experiment, French scientist Bichat writes: "I observed that at the end of a period in the dissecting rooms, my wind frequently took on an odor identical with the odor exhaled by decomposing corpses. Now, I ascertained that it was the skin as much as the lungs that absorbed the smelling molecules at that time, in the following way: I held my nostrils and fixed a fairly long pipe that went from my mouth out of the window, to enable me to breathe outside air. And what did I

find? After I had remained one hour in a small dissecting theater, next to two very fetid corpses, my wind produced an odor very similar to theirs."

For most people we know, however, food choice has to be the main determiner of fart behavior and character. Milk deserves a special note. For the many people with lactase deficiency, drinking milk is a sure-fire way to generate a lot of sure fires. One lactase-deficient 28-year-old man, described by Dr. Michael D. Levitt in "Studies of a Flatulent Patient" (*New England Journal of Medicine*, July 29, 1976), farted 70 times in four hours after two days of drinking only milk, mocking the average for a man of his age, a paltry 14 times per day.

Dr. Levitt has more fun stories to tell, such as the time a surgeon who, while cauterizing a rectal polyp, ignited a large fart (evidently with a high hydrogen content), causing an explosion which blew him back into the wall and ripped open six inches of the patient's colon. Fortunately, both doctor and patient survived.

As Spike Milligan writes in *Adolf Hitler: My Part in his Downfall*, the flammable potential of farts provided British soldiers with untold hours of amusement in the barracks of World War II, when fart-lighting contests (and contests to see who could best impersonate Groucho Marx with his genitals) were favored pastimes. Flammability in mind, Dr. Theodor Rosebury hypothesizes that had mammalian evolution placed the anus closer to the mouth, smoking would never have become popular.

The minor fire hazard is really the sole physical danger of farting. More attention by far has been paid to the physical dangers of *not* farting, and, as is to be expected, some of the finest scholars in history have come out firmly on the side of expulsion.

In 400 B.C., Hippocrates wrote, "It is best when wind passes without noise, but it is better that flatulence should pass even thus than it should be retained." In the eleventh century, the doctors at the enormously influential medical school in Salerno, Italy wrote that those who hold it in "risk dropsy, convulsions, vertigo, and fright-

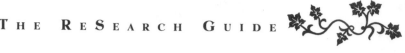

ful colics." Later, Montaigne observed "God alone knows how many times our bellies, by the refusal of one single fart, have brought us to the door of an agonizing death." Sir Thomas More felt strongly enough about the matter to express his sentiments in verse. The translation, from the Latin, is by Sir John Harington:

> "To breake a little wind, sometimes one's life doth save,
>
> For want of vent behind, some folk their ruin have:
>
> A powre it hath therefore, of life, and death expresse:
>
> A king can cause no more, a cracke [fart] doth do no lesse."

But the historical figure most spooked by the supposed dangers of holding 'em in was Emperor "I," Claudius of Rome, who ruled 41-54 A.D. After hearing a story about a man who nearly died as a result of his flatal modesty, he considered issuing an imperial edict specifically allowing farts at the dinner table.

Claudius's decree never made it out, but there actually have been some laws, formal customs at least, regarding farts. One of these was practiced in Britain up until the late 1800's. To sustain tenure on their estates, landholders had to appear every year at around New Year's in front of the lord or king who officially owned the land, and perform an involved ritual that included jumping up and farting in mid-air. Meanwhile, in France in the 1400's, prostitutes crossing the bridge of Montluc into town to start work were required to let a fart as a bridge toll. The origin of the fart as a form of payment probably goes back to pagan beliefs that bodily functions are tokens of living things, and that sacrificing living things appeases malevolent spirits.

Once we get into the less formalized area of Manners, tables turn on the fart. Etiquette books, when they mention farts at all (many don't), generally recommend against them, old English ones using quaint phrases like "Beware of thy hinder parts from gunblasting" and "Don't fire your sternguns." In the Victorian era, proper ladies would swoon dramatically if they farted audibly.

Europeans, however, seem to be more casual even than the rest of the world. During the slave trade, Ghanans were appalled at the Dutch colonists' free farting habits, regarding farting in the presence of strangers as extremely insulting. In China, Taoism forbade farting, along with spitting and weeping, in a northward direction. In most Arab nations, voiding wind was traditionally considered a great indecency. More recently, in our own country, "Miss Manners," displaying a genius for circumlocutory delicacy (as well as a nice sense of humor), writes, in 1983:

> *"Unacceptable Noises.* Miss Manners does not plan to mention them, chiefly because they are unmentionable, but you all know who you are. What they are. At any rate, these are noises that are acknowledged by neither the noisemaker nor the noise recipient, because socially they do not exist. The practice of staring hard at the person next to you when, for instance, your own stomach has given off a loud rumble, is therefore to be condemned on grounds of etiquette as well as morals."

In a later book, Miss Manners relates an illustrative story about Queen Elizabeth. The Queen and another chief of state were reviewing troops on horseback when a loud fart came from her direction. She immediately apologized for her horse's having broken wind, and her host graciously brushed it off but then added that had she not mentioned it, he would have actually thought the horse had done it.

One interesting exception to the "farting is impolite everywhere" rule is the Yanomami people of Venezuela. Among the Yanomami, farting is used as a greeting. Undoubtedly the "Miss Manners" of the Yanomami would recommend that, should a polite individual be unable to fart upon meeting a friend, the both of them should simply pretend that the fart did occur, and continue on as if it actually happened, never acknowledging otherwise. One's heart goes out to the unfortunate Yanomami child who doesn't fit in socially and has low self-esteem because his intestines are unable to produce enough gas.

Joseph Pujol, the Fartiste may have been the most successful at his craft, but he wasn't the first. St. Augustine and Montaigne both wrote about posterior trumpeters who could actually play melodies, and, in London in 1787, an anonymous author published a pamphlet entitled "An Essay Upon Wind" which included the story of "the Farting Blacksmith" of Kirkeaton, Yorkshire. The blacksmith could play tunes anally, and actually died in mid-rendition of his famous "Blow High, Blow Low" from popping a blood vessel. As contemporary scholar Eric Partridge notes, during this time, "the ability to play tunes by skillfully regulating and controlling one's windy expressions was regarded as. . .a most joyous and praiseworthy form of wit."

The same or a similar underground pamphlet to the one Partridge mentions, "The Benefit of Farting Explained, Wrote in Spanish by Don Fart in Hando, translated into English by Obadiah Fizle" had its tenth printing in 1722, indicating substantial popularity. But prudish attitudes have always fought against candor, despite popular sentiment. Some fairly recent editions of Chaucer's *Canterbury Tales* omit the farting and bunghole-branding part of the "Miller's Tale," its climax, rendering the whole story a meaningless buildup with no punch line. The British Greek scholar Dr. Gilbert Murray insisted on translating "to fart" as "to blow one's nose," destroying the jokes that begin Aristophanes' *The Clouds*.

Dr. Murray had a tough choice, though. Finding a proper word to use when describing the action directly, when no beating around the bush will do, has posed difficulties. Recently the medical establishment has wisely begun accepting *fart* as a proper term, following the word's recent weakening as an obscenity. More obscure and therefore more "polite" synonyms, which people might not understand (thereby assuring total politeness), are *flatulate*, *crepitate*, and *eructate*. Another is *pass wind*, and I'm still wondering if the folks responsible for a cassette I spied in the New Age music section of a record store, containing music ostensibly recorded by a group called "Past Wind," aren't just secretly making fun of the whole genre.

Fart facts and fictions:

- It takes only 10 minutes for swallowed air to make its way down to the large intestine, meaning that, as fart expert Mike Kimball puts it, "Breakfast's food (and the gas it generates) gets there the same time as air from lunch."
- Farts-to-be can sometimes actually be *seen* as dark cloudy areas on X-rays of the pelvis.
- In Luther's time, the morality plays often contained stage directions such as "Here Satan letteth a fart." Luther himself, however (the rebel), insisted that the Devil actually fled from farting, and on numerous occasions dreamt of chasing the Devil away in just such a manner.
- Apprentice baseball umpires are taught to never fart on the field thereby losing the catcher's respect.
- Morticians vigorously massage the corpse's lower abdomen to release any trapped, newly-generated gas. In the past, neglect of this procedure has resulted in the departed's farting during open-casket viewings.

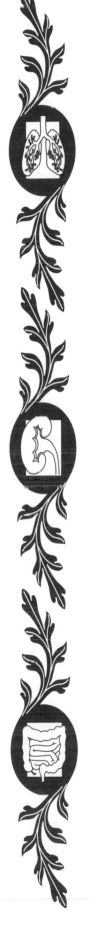

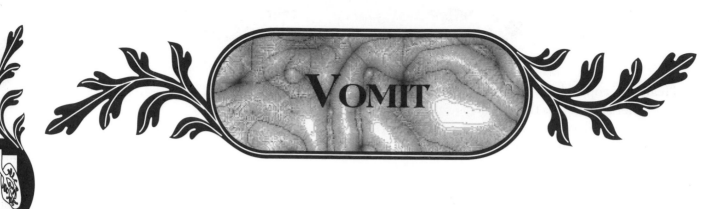

VOMIT

Blowing It
BLOW CHUNKS/CHUNKY/LUNCH/CHOW/DIN-DIN/ BEETS/DOUGHNUTS/GROCERIES/FOAM (IF BEER)

Religious/Reverential
KNEEL BEFORE THE PORCELAIN THRONE, BOW DOWN BEFORE THE PORCELAIN GOD, WORSHIP AT THE PORCELAIN ALTAR, PRAY TO THE PORCELAIN, MAKE FOOD OFFERINGS TO THE CHINA GODS, OFFER SACRIFICE TO RALPH

Modified Vocalization
TECHNICOLOR YAWN/YODEL, LIQUID LAUGH/SCREAM, SHOUT AT YOUR SHOES, LAUGH AT THE CARPET, YELL AT THE GROUND, SING YOUR LUNCH, SING TO THE SINK

Onomatopoetry
HEAVE, GACK, YAK, PUKE, BARF, RETCH, WOOF, YUKE, BRACK, GAG, BOOT, CHUCK, URP

Your Old Pals
RALPH, EARL, MEET MY FRIENDS RALPH AND EARL, TALK TO RALPH/EARL/HUEY ON THE BIG WHITE/ PORCELAIN TELEPHONE, YELL/CALL FOR HUEY, CALL EARL'S

General Cleverness
JOIN THE DANIEL BOONE CLUB (BACKPACKER LINGO: "YOU SHOOT YOUR LUNCH"), BRING IT UP FOR A VOTE, ROUND-TRIP MEAL TICKET, READ THE TOILET, FEED THE FISH (IN THE HUDSON), MAKE A (TECHNICOLOR) TRIBUTE TO DISNEY, LIQUIDATE YOUR ASSETS, GO TO BOOT CAMP, THE BIG SPIT

Origins
CHUCK A PIZZA, SPEW SPUDS, DELIVER STREET/ SIDEWALK PIZZA, CHEW YOUR FRIES SOME MORE, WOOF YOUR COOKIES, LOSE/LEAVE LUNCH, TOSS YOUR TACOS, SPILL THE GROCERIES, FLASH YOUR HASH

Transportation
DRIVE THE PORCELAIN BUS, SELL CARS, SELL A BUICK, BUICK, REVERSE GEARS, RIDE THE REGURGITRON, CALL BUICKS

Biology
FEED YOUR YOUNG, CALL DINOSAURS, CALL TO THE SEALS, BARK AT ANTS

Scientific and Technical
REVERSE GUT, REVERSE DIARRHEA, PROTEIN SPILL, NEGATIVE CHUG, REVERSE PERISTALSIS, UN-EAT, NEGATIVE CHUG, REVERSE DRINK, VECTOR SPEW, ANTIPERISTALSIS, LOSE WEIGHT

The Sporting Scene
HURL, POWER BOOT, CATCH IT ON THE REBOUND, LATERAL COOKIE TOSS

Polite
DISGORGE, REGURGITATE, UP-CHUCK, SPEW, CHUNDER, PARBREAKE, OOPS

Home and Garden Improvement
CLEAN HOUSE, PLANT BEETS, FERTILIZE THE SIDE-WALK, DECORATE PAVEMENT

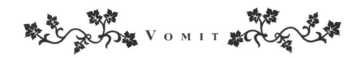
Healthy people don't throw up regularly, so, unlike other substances this book discusses, vomit cannot be considered a product of the body's normal functioning. But nearly all of us can recall at least a few episodes of involuntary food review, and in my experience, people who like talking about the normal bodily functions also like to talk about vomiting. I've attended many social gatherings where swapping vomit anecdotes has fueled lively conversations among people who otherwise don't share many interests.

But there's more to vomit than people's barf stories. Vomiting has a history. During Roman times, public vomiting in special buildings was an activity of the very rich. Later, vomiting came to be associated with demonic possession and witchcraft. Also, vomit relates to some open scientific questions. For example, although progress is being made, science still cannot fully explain nausea and disgust. We still don't know why disgust, which is as fundamental a reaction as fear or happiness, operates over such a limited domain, and we've only recently discovered some of the basic mechanisms of motion discomfort.

People, Places, and Puking (Survey)

Vomiting Section

When was the last time you threw up?

No surprises here. Many respondents answer imprecisely, as in "last Spring" or "in high school," but my feeling is that with more accuracy, answers would fall into a pretty normal distribution against a log time scale (like less than one week ago, one to two weeks ago, two to four weeks ago, four to eight weeks ago, and so on), with the peak at a bit less than one year ago (the 32 to 64 weeks ago bin, using the log 2 week scale). With the accuracy I had, the numbers looked like this: 5% had barfed within the last week, 15% had last thrown up between one and eight weeks ago, 27% last vomited between eight weeks and one year ago, 26% had most recently puked between one and five years ago, and 5% have not booted at all during the past five years. 9% say they can't remember or that it was a very long time ago, "many many moons ago" as one young woman puts it, and one iron-stomached student who must have been a low-maintenance infant, claims that she has never thrown up.

The more recent barfers, who are generally the more frequent ones as well, tend not to give specific dates, but many of those who seldom vomit can pinpoint their last regurgitation with confidence. One man in his thirties answers, "February 1973." A writer in his forties replies, "1963." A teen answers, "In third grade."

What were the surrounding circumstances?

Despite the word "circumstances," many people answer with locations only: "bathroom," "in the street," and the like. Even so, a full 37% of respondents point to alcohol poisoning, making circumstances that lead to it by far the top category for this question. 5% buffer the admission by mentioning foods that accompanied the

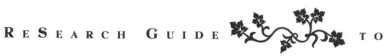

drug beverages, as in, "green clams and Ripple" and, "drinking and bad party food," but most lay the blame on demon drink alone, with answers such as, "inebriation," "a drunken binge," "hung over," "entirely too much beer," and, "I had drunk rather heavily." One young man boasts, "drank a case of beer and a bottle of tequila." Another generalizes, "I basically only puke when I get disgustingly drunk, when I puke lots." A young woman shares, "Drunk, at home, into a 9" x 9" square casserole dish."

6% mention parties, either with or without alcohol. For one young man, it was at a "buddy's bachelor party." Another succumbed to "Four hours of straight rum and gin drinking at a card party."

Extended illness (as opposed to food poisoning), most often stomach flu, defines the next most numerous group, with 18% of respondents. Another 11% blame food poisoning, pointing to such culprits as "bad fish," kim chee, and empanadas. A former Gainesville resident warns, "Don't order the Big Skeeter Special."

10% say they were in the bathroom. One woman explains, "I was in the bathroom on the toilet, threw up in the bathtub." A political-conflict minded young man relates, "Shower. I was brushing my tongue and I crossed that lingual DMZ and a Nation's burger came up."

3% were camping or traveling when they last yakked. Another 3% can't remember the circumstances, and 3% more threw up as a result of taking prescription drugs. A male grad student describes his bad experience with Tylenol 3, which contains codeine. The doctor who had attended to his badly cut finger warned him that the painkiller would aggravate motion sickness, but he took the bus to work the following day anyway. He managed to step off the bus and make it to a low cement wall before losing it.

2% had ingested hallucinogenic mushrooms the last time they vomited. Another 2% say they hurled out of nervousness, and another 2% vomited from overeating. Other circumstances people mention include "Just finished having sex" and "In full daylight at a Fleetwood Mac concert."

Do you throw up often? About how often?

64% answer that they don't throw up often while only 5% say they do. Of respondents who give hard numbers, most claim to vomit between once every two months and once a year. 1% vomit more often than semiweekly, 4% vomit between semiweekly and semimonthly, and 8% vomit once a year to once every five years. 9% simply say they vomit very infrequently, 4% claim to have vomited only a few times as adults or ever, and 3% maintain that they "never" vomit or haven't since childhood.

8% say they only vomit when they're drunk and 5% claim to vomit only when they're sick. Three respondents say they used to vomit often. One did it daily when he was taking Navane. Another writes, "I used to throw up four to five times a year due to poor digestive system. I guess the California air has done me good." Finally, two respondents claim to vomit annually—one "Every Spring" and the other "Every St. Pat's Day."

Have you ever made yourself throw up? Why?

People split evenly on this one, with 46% each Yes and No. Meanwhile, 4% have tried but failed. The most common motivation, with 15%, is to avoid a hangover or to hasten the inevitable during alcoholic inebriation. One young man notes that under these circumstances, the task is not difficult. Meanwhile, a hard-partying dude of 25 offers a related but different motivation: to enable himself "to drink some more."

The second-place reason, accounting for 10%, is to relieve nausea, illness, or a sick feeling not related to alcohol consumption. In these situations, as with drinking, great effort is often unnecessary. One young man writes, "No, but once I realized there were maggots in my pasta and I kind of wanted to throw up, so I did."

6%, most of them women, have thrown up to empty their stomachs, with another 1% explicitly saying that they do it to control their weight. One teen explains, "Yeah! Because I was too full! And because I didn't like the food!" A 22-year-old gives the curious explanation, "Yes—sick from eating too much—blood vessels above my eyes popped."

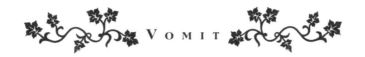

The 4% who have unsuccessfully tried to vomit give various motivations: to relieve nausea, to mitigate alcohol poisoning, and to empty the stomach prior to taking hallucinogenic mushrooms. One young man who has never tried making himself boot doubts if he ever could.

2% mention having vomited to avoid having to go to school. The remaining respondents give a wide assortment of unique rationales, including to puke on an enemy in fifth grade, to be able to continue dancing, to avoid possible food poisoning after eating green-tinged luncheon meat, for pure experimentation as a kid, to expel disagreeable medicine, drugs, or accidentally-ingested hydrogen peroxide, "fraternity bullshit," and, according to a 37-year-old programmer, "Just for the fun of it. Just for the taste of it."

What was the most embarrassing place you ever threw up?

8% answer that they have never thrown up anyplace embarrassing or, as a 35-year-old musician expresses it, have "always made it to Mr. Porcelain." A 24-year-old writes, "I have never been embarrassed to throw up." Most others have not been so lucky.

11% vomited with discomfiture in or out of cars or vans, including a date's car, the grandparents' car, and a taxicab. One unfortunate threw up in his own car, all over himself, while driving.

8% had the humiliating experience of barfing at school, including in the lunchroom, on a plant, and outside the main (high school) building. Two threw up in math class. One, now an occupational health specialist, puts it like this [abridged]: "The night before the last day of class my freshman year, I partied really hard. I drank a lot of tequila (to this day, the smell of tequila makes me ill). The next morning I felt like barfing, but I didn't want to miss the very last day of class. I figured that if I had a good breakfast, the sick feeling would go away. Not even! [Toward the end of class] I felt worse and worse. I was starting to salivate. Then the clock struck the hour. I started to get up, and felt this surge in my stomach, but I managed to hold it in. I

still had to get out of the room. The door was at the back, I was towards the front, and a line of people was hampering my progress to the exit. I was almost there when a second surge hit. I covered my mouth, but a little got out and some went zinging through my nose. I think it hit the person in front of me. Then a huge contraction hit my stomach. I dove for the garbage can and puked an incredible amount into it. I looked up and saw the rest of my classmates leave the room. One guy asked me if I was all right. I told him I felt great."

Another 8% had puked at parties. One young man of 20 remembers that it had happened "at a party where I was trying to hook this beautiful girl." A young man who describes himself as a Libra recalls, "Once, at a party, after several beers and bong loads, I suddenly got the spins and found I needed to boot. Much to my chagrin, the bathroom was locked, so I threw up on the door. Fortunately, a friend vacuumed it up for me."

7% were most embarrassed by vomiting on others, including roommates, friends, mothers, waiters, boyfriends, and "two women on a train in Portugal." 5% mention having thrown up on sidewalks, streets, curbs, or pavement. Another 5% puked on or out of buses and trains or on train platforms. One of these wound up clearing an entire subway car as a result.

4% mention having thrown up on themselves or their own clothes, including a lawyer who threw up into his shorts while sitting on the toilet. 3% recall throwing up in parking lots or garages. Another 3% recall yakking in restaurants, including "Two feet short of the sink at Cantor's [delicatessen in Los Angeles]," and another 3% lost it on airplanes, including a small six-seat airplane containing several people known to the victim.

2% mention bars or night clubs, including one young man who upchucked on the bar itself, as he writes, "in front of a bartendress I fancied." Another 2% threw up during dates, and 2% more hurled on carpets, including one teen who writes, "A friend's carpet (white carpet) — all over — and I'd been eating chocolate cake."

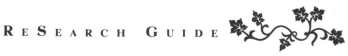

Other embarrassing vomit locales include a police station, a friend's window screen, a Thanksgiving dinner, the Worlds Of Fun amusement park in Kansas City, a public pool, a trash can at the Special Olympics' opening ceremonies, a tent, a front porch, a front lawn, a stairwell, an airplane jetway, a boat, and a dock in Hawaii. Two more unique locations deserve the participants' full descriptions. First, a woman of 22 answers, "In bed—gagged while giving blowjob—you can guess the rest. I covered it up pretty well." Finally, a 32-year-old man recalls, "I once pigged out on oranges immediately after my match at a wrestling match and promptly barfed them into a towel that I then stuck under my chair. The next wrestler then sat down hot and sweaty after his match, and before I could stop him he used the towel to wipe his face."

Ever "chug" and then "power boot"? How far did it go? Did you win? Who did?

5% indicate that they don't understand the terms this question uses. The expressions refer to swallowing beer and then intentionally projectile-vomiting it for maximum distance in a contest. The sport is particularly popular among scholar-athletes at universities.

Most participants say they have not chugged and power booted, but 5% say they have, including a 21-year-old male student who answers the questions, "Fuck yeah! Quite a ways. No. Someone else," an apologetic teenager who writes, "Yes, never was good at it. Always lost," and a triumphant 22-year-old who answers, "Yes. Many meters. Of course. Me," and then adds in pencil-breaking heavy printing, "My nickname is RALPH!"

A 20-year-old answers that he once "saw someone 'boot' six feet," a lucky occasion in the opinion of a 25-year-old grad student who writes, "Never experienced this, but I would love to *watch* a competition."

A 26-year-old programmer recounts, "No, but two friends from high school, Blake Traister and Even Eustis, had a 'quarters 'til you yak' contest. Even 'won' and was ecstatic when Blake threw

up beer all over him."

Power booting has its detractors, however. A 35-year-old man exclaims, "Not a frat guy, no!" A 20-year-old woman "Philosophy turned Rhetoric major who intends on making films" writes, "Pu-leease. Frat boy fixations. I value my health."

Finally, a precocious young woman of 18 answers, "Not recently."

What is your favorite food to throw up (if such a preference has ever occurred to you)?

36% say they have no preference, 5% say they've never thought about it, and 3% simply say they don't know, but most of the rest of the respondents, it turns out, have clear and specific preferences when it comes to yakking material. Few foods receive more than one vote, however, making our taste in vomit as individual and special as our taste in music or art.

Some foods do have plural followings, though. Pizza easily tops the list with 6% of the vote, all male. Some participants even specify toppings. A 19-year-old computer technician favors green peppers and onions, a 22-year-old "beer drinker" prefers pizza "with greasy pork sausage," and a 29-year-old attorney votes for pepperoni. Pizza's only opponent is a 31-year-old woman who opines, "liquid [is] much better than pizza," reflecting not only the apparent male preference for pizza, but also a female preference for throwing up liquid foods. Of the 8% total who list liquids, including soup, orange juice, milk, water, Coke, beer, and liquids in general, most are women—especially significant, given the sample's male bias. From these results, it seems likely that in general, women prefer regurgitating liquids while men prefer to throw up pizza.

Meanwhile, 4% favor spaghetti, macaroni and cheese, or other pasta. 3% like to throw up peas best, and 2% each prefer corn and bananas. One corn advocate explains her choice with, "I like to throw up corn because it stays whole."

Single votes honor foods such as chicken, beans, beef stew, mushrooms, potatoes, mince, ice cream, eggs, oatmeal, "something sweet," Mexi-

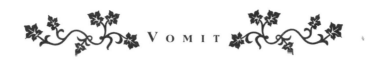

can food, fish, chicken pot pies, hot dogs, spinach, and firm strawberry Jell-O. Sometimes these votes come with explanations such as "Hot dog—you can see the casing separated from the meat," "Spinach when it's way down in the stomach," and "Mexican—it tastes as good coming up as it did going down." A former bulimic explains that "Among bulimics, it's well-known that ice cream after a binge makes it all come up easily."

Several people mention vomit anti-preferences. Two say they particularly dislike vomiting spicy foods. Another mentions orange juice. A 30-year-old explains, "I don't like to boot foods that I like; I have an aversion to eating foods that I have puked, so I don't want to puke foods I like."

3% simply say they don't ever like vomiting, well-represented by the 31-year-old woman who writes, "Eww—I *hate* barfing." In a similar vein, the 20-year-old rhetoric major and future filmmaker answers, "Pea soup. No, just kidding. *Nothing*, you obscure, sick-minded creature! Stomach acids aren't exactly a culinary delight." (Cheese-lovers would disagree.)

Finally, a 22-year-old dance teacher answers simply, "something substantial," and a 38-year-old researcher notes, "seems to me that whenever I vomit there is some trace of a tomato product."

Ever make anyone else throw up? How? Why?

58% say they have not done this and 5% answer more conservatively, saying they don't know, can't recall having done so, or that they doubt it. A 24-year-old working in sports promotions answers, "No, but I'd like to."

4% induced vomiting in sick, drunk, or drugged friends or relatives. Where specified, this was with a finger down the throat.

3% made others vomit by throwing up themselves, presumably unintentionally. Another 3% did it by serving them alcoholic beverages or drinking with them. A male 27-year-old writes, "Well, once I gave a bottle of Scotch to a girl to share, and you know, she lost it." A 22-year-old fellow answers the questions, "Yes. Beer pressure. I wanted to, she was cute." A teenage lad jokes "I chugged with him. He lost both the contest and

its contents."

A 28-year-old man made another guy ralph by putting his hand in dog feces. A spunky 16-year-old woman did it by punching the person in the stomach. Another young woman made her brother vomit by sneezing on him. Finally, an unemployed 22-year-old claims she caused nausea by telling a bad joke, and a 35-year-old musician answers, "Just with my music!"

What literally nauseates you?

I had hoped that the word "literally" in the question would discourage answers like "liberals" or "homosexuals," but I should have known better. A lot of respondents used this question to "literally" run up the flagpole and air out all the personal, petty, dirty axes to grind that they have sitting in their closets. Into this category I put such answers as "beat-type music," "White male European reactions to fear," "people who don't drop LSD," Phil Collins, religion, homosexuals, "sorority bimbos talking about modeling," abortion, liberals, "chicks who don't party," fat women, "anyone anal retentive," pedophilia, "men with too much cologne," "women with excess perfume," police violence, presidential candidates, panhandling, suffering, chauvinism, sexism, Rush Limbaugh, Republicans, President Bush, and tasteless people. While I detest some of the sentiments here expressed and agree with or are indifferent to others, they all disappoint me by missing the intent of the question.

9% claim that nothing or not much nauseates them, including one assured young man who answers the question with, "Nothing. I mean that."

For the rest, vomit itself is the clear least-favorite. 24% of respondents answer that vomit, the smell of vomit, seeing another person vomit, etc. nauseated them. A biology grad student gets nauseated by, "Other people's barf. Animal barf isn't so bad." For a young programmer, it's "cleaning up warm throw-up."

Next, with 11%, is flesh and blood: innards, blood, meat, spoiled meat, dead animals, dead bodies, open flesh, operations, blood and guts movies, etc. Another respondent specifically men-

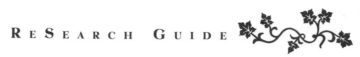

tions eating fatty meat, and another one lists open heart surgery.

7% mention feces or fecal smells, including "shit floating in pool," "pig poo," "fresh baby shit," and "shit with maggots," with another 1% mentioning "latrine smells" in general. 5% mention bus or car trips. 3% mention spitting or slobber. 2% each mention bad smells of any sort, amusement park rides, urine or urine smells, maggots, flu or germs, pus-filled zits, and too much coffee or tea early in the morning.

Several participants say they're nauseated by various foods, including cheese, mustard and mayonnaise, runny eggs, and "bad fish." For others, it's even just the smells of foods, particularly of clams, hops, and fried eggplant. One more respondent lists, "soggy food stuck in kitchen sink."

Non-food, non-excrement odors also make the list, including the smells of sulfur, gasoline, trash dumpsters, cat spray, and female genitalia, the last being mentioned by a 22-year-old male student. An 18-year-old woman, meanwhile, lists "cum taste."

One young woman mentions pregnancy as nauseous. Another, for the same physiological reasons, lists birth control pills.

Assorted other nauseators that participants list include boluses of chewed food, used tampons, castor oil and root beer (consumed together at a doctor's request, to "flush out" the system before a kidney exam), hordes of insects, overeating, people of casual hygiene, hearing two people having sex and groaning, animal experimentation, mucus, and, inevitably, "this survey."

Are you susceptible to "motion discomfort"? Where?

41% say they do not experience motion discomfort. One knowledgeable eighteen-year-old answers, "No—I know some reliable pressure points." For the rest, motion can cause nausea, nearly always the motion of a motor vehicle. 33% get sick in cars or vans, 8% mention buses, 3% mention airplanes, and 1% mention trains. 9% say it happens while reading, and 6% say it happens in the mountains or on winding mountain roads.

The breadth of answers shows the range of people's sensitivities. One teen answers, "Bus, cars, anything with more than two wheels." A bit more rugged are the two 25-year-olds who answer, "Moving vehicles without sources of fresh air," and "Reading in winding mountain trails aboard a bus with no ventilation." And some people remain unmoved in all but a very specific set of circumstances, like the 17-year-old woman who answers, "Only when blindfolded and in constant motion," or the 30-year-old man who writes, "When riding [in cars], and on days when the sun is low in the sky and bright light slants in at a very low elevation."

9% mention boats or ships. One Canadian-born 37-year-old who has not thrown up since 1973 answers, "Boats but I no boot."

Other locations and settings of mention include roller coasters, the "teacups" at Disneyland, swings, and underwater dives.

Any major events make you throw up (weddings, PhD orals, PhD anals)?

I was surprised by how few participants seriously answer that this has happened to them: only 6%. Meanwhile, 65% answer No, 1% say "Not that I remember," and 1% just put a question mark. A few gave joke answers à la "What literally nauseates you?": the 1980 Presidential election, sorority meetings, etc. 3% took the bait and indicated that their PhD anal examinations had caused them to vomit.

Others mention throwing up after running a cross-country race in high school, at someone else's wedding after drinking a lot, when visiting Mom at the hospital after an accident, and at Christmastime.

A teenage woman hypothesizes, "If someone gave me a check-up at a gynecologist's I would." Finally, a 26-year-old man writes, "No, but I gotta pinch many liquid loaves when I'm nervous."

Ever throw up into your mouth and then swallow it again?

38% of respondents say they've done this, while 46% say they haven't. Only 2%, however, have

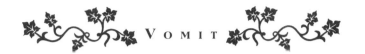

anything nice to say about the experience: one 26-year-old fellow writes, "No, though I wish I had," while another answers, "Belching—yummy . . . . I enjoy belching up non-spicy foods."

The rest seem to view vomiturition more dimly. Various Noes respond, "No, but I fear it," "No, but I probably wouldn't be hungry again for a while," and, from a 20-year-old who says he likes Dungeons and Dragons: "NOPE! THAT WOULD MAKE ME THROW IT UP AGAIN! AAAIIIGH!" Two Yesses report, "Just a little—major nasty!" and "Yes, it's kind of gross 'cause it comes back out again." One man answers, "No, I'm not that type of a boy." Another asks, "Isn't that what happened to Jimi [Hendrix]?" Two frank young men explain, "Some, but I never chew," and, "Once, but I spit it out after a while."

A few people give the names they use to describe this set of actions: mini-puke, barfy burps, belching (a nonstandard usage), ajidas, and McPhailing.

Ever throw up into your hands and then eat it again, like this kid next to me on the school bus once did (the memory haunts me to this day)?

73% answer No, 3% answer Yes, 4% express distaste ("Ugh!," "yuck," etc.), 2% say they've seen dogs or cats do it, and 2% claim that they were the ones I saw on the bus. One young man who may have thought I could be an old classmate answers, "Yes, at Merrick Woods Day School when I was 5."

Two participants apparently like the idea, answering, "No, but that's a Kool thought," and "No, but I'd like to see it done." Others share memories of their own, with "No, but we've seen others do this," "No, but there was a week in school when four of the five days a different kid in class threw up," and, "No, but I saw a girl throw up into her hands on a bus, and her gum was floating in it (my haunting memory)."

For others, however, the query provokes questioning and even distrust. One 27-year-old businessman writes, "I don't do this, I haven't done this, and I'm suspicious." Finally, a 20-year-old

student asks, "What's this fascination with *eating* repulsive excretions? Do you like sushi?"

The Psychology of Disgust

Unlike love or sadness or anger, the emotion of disgust doesn't often inspire people to write sonnets or fight duels, but nevertheless it is considered a basic human emotion, with its own characteristic facial expression and physiological manifestation (nausea). But it stands apart from other emotions for a couple of reasons: it's quite specific, as basic emotions go, and it's probably uniquely human. These two aspects make its origins and exact function quite a mystery.

Why should an entire emotion, with all the complicated neurological machinery that has to come with it, be hardwired into our brains to deal with such a limited set of circumstances? There are many things we don't eat, but only a few of them actually disgust us; nightshade leaves and toadstools don't disgust us at all, for example, despite their poison. Also, one culture's disgusting can be another's delicacy; some cultures view lobsters and cheeses the way we view greasy grimy gopher guts and marinated monkey meat. Furthermore, disgust only appears in humans above the age of four, even though children under four are the ones whose inexperience and small size make them more likely to eat dangerous things and more susceptible to their effects.

There's a lot we don't know about disgust, but, fortunately, disgust (defined operationally as "revulsion at the prospect of oral incorporation of an object"), is a subject of scientific research. One study, described in Volume 50 of the *Journal of Personality and Social Psychology* (1986), involved several experiments. For one, subjects were asked to rate the appeal of fruit juice before and after either a dried sterilized cockroach or a plastic birthday candle holder was stirred in. Another experiment had subjects rate the appeal of a normal square of fudge, followed by pieces of the same fudge shaped to resemble either muffins or

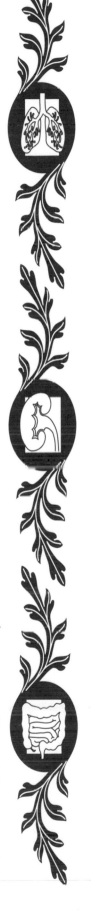

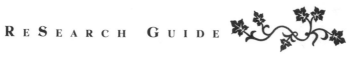

feces. In a third experiment, subjects were presented with a rubber sink stopper and a rubber imitation vomit, ("purchased in a novelty store," the article explains), and asked to rate their inclination to hold each between their lips for ten seconds.

The authors of this study concluded that Americans endow things they find disgusting with actual "magical" properties, according to laws of sympathetic magic described by anthropologists. These laws hold that good or evil powers will pass from source objects into other objects they touch, resemble, or are associated with. Belief in sympathetic magic has traditionally been considered characteristic only of non-technocentric cultures.

What we learn from the experiments themselves, however, is that doing research in psychology can provide us with both a greater understanding of our minds and yucks aplenty.

Some of the other experiments proposed and conducted by our nation's top disgust researchers, most notably Paul Rozin of the University of Pennsylvania and April Fallon of Pennsylvania Medical College, are as follows:

• Ask people to rate the appeal of soup served in a regular bowl, in a new dog dish, in a used, cleaned dog dish, in a new bed pan, stirred by a new fly swatter, and stirred by a used, cleaned fly swatter. Ask them to rate the relative appeals of glasses of juice after seeing sterilized, dead cockroaches and plastic birthday candle holders (the control) stirred in. Finding: further evidence linking disgust with belief in sympathetic magic.

• Ask kids of various ages to eat cookies sprinkled with colored sugar or what the experimenter presents as ground-up grasshopper. Ask them to drink juice after immersing in it a sterilized, dried grasshopper or an (apparently) used comb. Finding: sensitivity to perceived contamination by disgusting substances increases steadily between the ages of 4 and 12, and then levels off.

• Ask people to rate the appeal of a normal bowl of soup, one they've just spat into, and one they've spat some chewed food into.

Finding: one's own saliva becomes "disgusting" once it leaves one's body.

• Ask people who like strong cheeses to distinguish between two vials containing identical decay scents, claiming that one contains cheese and the other feces. Then tell the subject that the one selected as cheese is actually feces, and observe the reaction. Finding: people's conception of an object, rather than its sensory properties alone, determines disgust.

Some scientists have argued that the disgust reaction grew out of the time when our vegetarian ancestors started eating meat, a fundamental switch that resulted from their inability to reliably obtain adequate nutrition from vegetable sources alone. Meat-eating is new to our species, and we still feel ambivalent toward it; we crave meat for its nutrients and yet are repelled by it as something that, through nearly all of our evolution, we were programmed to never consider ingesting. Many vestiges of our vegetarian past remain, in addition to disgust. Every culture accepts very few animal species as food, when compared with the number available, and vegetarianism, usually with some religious significance, shows up in cultures around the world. Moreover, traditional recipes often disguise meat's animal origin, further suggesting that we aren't wholly comfortable with our new dietary habit.

Others have taken the theory further, suggesting that feces, particularly the feces of humans and mammalian carnivores, stand above all other substances of animal origin as the "primary disgust substance." Feces are the first thing a child finds disgusting, beginning 3 to 6 years after toilet training, which the reaction may somehow hearken back to. Widespread use of the expression "Eat shit and die" attests to our strong fear of "orally incorporating" this particular substance. So the correct answer to the playground discussion question, "If you were up to your chin in shit and someone threw a bucket of puke at you, would you duck?" would, according to this view, be "No."

Many species regularly eat their own feces,

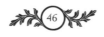

thereby getting to use nutrients generated in the intestines. Laboratory rats, for example, a species all scientists trust, eat fully half of their feces and seem to do just fine, so long as their Purina Rat Chow is free of carcinogenic additives. The reason we don't do this, and why other primates only do it occasionally, probably has to do with our living arrangements. The big danger from coprophagy is infection, the chances of which are greatly diminished when the individual consumes only his own feces, as is typically the case with coprophagous species. However, since we typically live closely with others, staying in the same area and defecating in a few fixed spots away from our "nests," it would be difficult to keep tabs on precisely whose logs in the logpile belonged to whom. So if we had, at some point in our evolution, started eating our feces, we'd have been eating everyone else's as well, and parasites and infections would have had a field day with the whole community. The risks outweigh the nutritional benefits.

The same goes for vomit. Given pool of vomit A, there was probably a good reason why A was thrown up in the first place, and since whatever agent it was that caused the regurgitation is probably still in here, another individual's re-eating A would not be advisable, no matter what the possible nutritional (or culinary) gain.

Why disgusting things don't simply occupy the "dangerous to eat" category in our minds, along with unidentified mushrooms and untreated acorns, is not completely clear. Rozin suggests that disgust also provides a strong mechanism through which to transmit food-related cultural values. The individual might start ignoring a taboo against a food considered dangerous but not disgusting if he discovers, upon breaking it once or twice, that there are no apparent, immediate harmful consequences, whereas if general properties of the tabooed material actually repel him, instinctively or through cultural conditioning, then he's much less likely to disregard the taboo in the face of any contrary evidence. In cases of disgust at harmful materials, this adaptation would have a greater benefit regarding those

which are infectious rather than simply toxic, because ingestion of an infectious agent can then affect the entire community, rather than just the individual (who, if he's stupid enough to be eating dangerous things, should probably be weeded out of the reproductive pool anyway). This fits in with our view; feces, vomit, and dead animals, the disgusting things, are more likely to be dangerous foods because of infectiousness rather than toxicity.

So we should be thankful for disgust. It may not inspire us to paint landscapes, launch ships or even bake cookies, but, like a mysterious, benevolent deity, it's always there to protect us. And so, when the time comes for it to work its sympathetic magic and we're suddenly inspired to launch our cookies, we'll say a prayer, a prayer to the porcelain, in thanks.

Waah! Motion Discomfort!

Airlines used to print "For Motion Discomfort" on their barf bags, but at some later time they must have realized that the plain white, plastic-lined sacks needed no explanation. Motion discomfort, motion sickness, airsickness, seasickness, carsickness, travel sickness—it's an infamous, familiar phenomenon whatever you call it, and it's older than the seafaring ancient Greeks, who coined an antecedent to our word "nausea" out of their word for ship.

Some adults have never experienced motion sickness, while others suffer from it frequently. Not surprisingly, recent work indicates that motion sensitivity has a genetic basis. More interesting, for trivia buffs at least, is a racial correlation: Asians get motion sickness more easily than do either Africans or Europeans. One explanation points to Asians' higher sensitivity to certain neurotransmitters. Motion sickness, which begins in the brain, may involve brain chemicals Asians

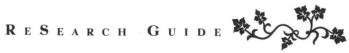

have a higher susceptibility to.

Motion sickness begins when what you see doesn't match what you feel, when visual signals telling you how you're moving conflict with messages coming from the balance center in your inner ear. A common situation occurs when you're inside a moving vehicle and your visual system, interpreting the vehicle's inside, "believes" that you're staying in one place. It can also happen the other way around; strong visual motion cues in a surround-screen theater on land can also cause nausea. Virtual Reality flight simulators, which fill operators' visual fields no matter where they look, are notorious nauseators.

In susceptible people, the eye/inner ear signal mismatch causes the brain to release increased quantities of the stress-related hormones epinephrine, norepinephrine, and vasopressin. These cause sweaty palms, headache, and other stress symptoms as well as stomach muscle convulsions that can lead to vomiting.

But we still don't know why this all has to happen in the first place. Why should we throw up just because we don't know if we're moving or not? Scientists aren't sure, but one theory explains that motion sickness is an evolutionary "mistake" related to our reaction to food poisoning. Early symptoms of food poisoning are dizziness and blurred vision, and to expel the poison food, we evolved a vomiting reaction triggered by these symptoms. But dizziness also results from the eye/inner ear signal mismatch we experience inside moving vessels. The theory proposes that the nausea reflex does not distinguish between these two causes of dizziness, food poisoning and mismatched motion cues, and initiates vomiting in both cases. Being tossed around in a boat mimics the early symptoms of food poisoning and causes an overgeneralized vomit reflex.

You can prevent motion sickness by taking a Dramamine or promethazine tablet or applying a scopolamine patch behind your ear, but these drugs can cause drowsiness and even, ironically, nausea. A recent study found ginger, long recommended by Chinese folk medicine, more effective than Dramamine at preventing motion sickness. Conspiracy theorists might note, correctly, that pharmaceutical companies would lose a lot of money if people started buying ginger and ginger candies instead of Dramamine and Transderm-Scop.

Another set of remedies focuses on acupuncture's P6, or the Nelguan point. Chinese acupuncturists have long treated nausea by inserting needles into the forearm skin between the tendons about an inch and a quarter from the wrist crease. Researchers have shown that applying a continuous electric current to this point also prevents nausea, and a battery-powered nausea-prevention wristband operating on this principle has recently been patented. Also, at least two companies now sell acupressure wristbands which press into the Nelguan point, but their usefulness has not yet been clearly differentiated from placebo effect.

There are also some simpler things you can do to prevent or diminish motion sickness: eat a small, low-fat, high-carbohydrate meal before the trip, keep your eyes on distant objects outside, don't move your head around much, and, most difficult of all, think about something other than how miserable you feel.

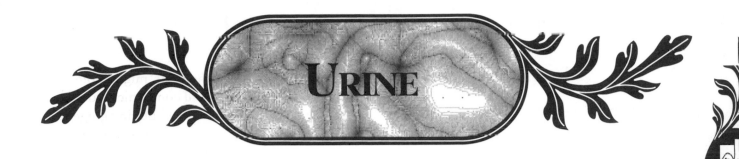

URINE

Urinate

MICTURATE, PASS WATER, PEE, TINKLE, PISS, SISSY, EASE YOURSELF, PICK A DAISY, MAKE ROOM FOR TEA, POINT PERCY AT THE PORCELAIN, SPEND A PENNY, SEE A MAN ABOUT A DOG, MAKE A PIT STOP, TURN YOUR BIKE AROUND, WEE, WHIZ, PIDDLE, DRAIN THE MAIN, STALE (LIVESTOCK), TAKE A LEAK/WHIZ/SQUIRT

Urine

PEE-PEE, NUMBER ONE, CHAMBER LYE

A Drunken Man who Urinates Under the Table on a Companion's Shoes

VICE-ADMIRAL OF THE NARROW SEAS (OLD BRITISH SLANG)

Parisian Men who Swallow Scum Obtained from Street Urinals

LES MANGEURS DU BLANC (THE EXPRESSION, ACCORDING TO BOURKE, ALSO REFERS TO PIMPS)

Urine analysis has long been useful for medical diagnosis, and as scientists have refined the process, it has become more informative than ever. The urine contains products of many of our bodies' chemical activities, providing a detailed history of what we've ingested, what toxins and mutagens we've been exposed to, and what our immune systems have been doing. The specific application of drug testing brought urinalysis into public focus several years ago.

Meanwhile, urine has a large following as a healing agent, and people throughout the world wash themselves with it and drink it in order to attain or maintain health.

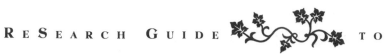

People, Places, and Peeing (Survey)

Urination Section

Do you get "Asparagus Pee"? "Coffee Pee"? "Neon Multivitamin Pee"?

The most widely produced, or at least most widely noticed, of these three unique urines is Neon Multivitamin Pee, with 28% of respondents saying they get it. The specially scented Coffee and Asparagus Pees run a close race for second with 23% for Coffee and 22% for Asparagus.

Regarding Neon Multivitamin Pee, described by one respondent as, "Major neon yellow, mon," a programmer notes, "Vitamin Pee also smells funky." Concerning Asparagus Pee, one woman exclaims, "People who don't notice this *amaze* me!" A young man clarifies that he gets Espresso Pee, and not simply Coffee Pee.

Several participants note other special urines they've experienced, including Beer Pee, Water Pee ("huge amounts of clear fluid"), Beet Pee, a urine with an unidentifiable, vaguely metallic odor, and a urine that was colored orange.

Ever time your pees? What's your "record"? Ever break a minute without beer?

48% say they don't time their pees, but 18% say they do, and give an impressive range of personal bests. The record high, an astonishing 2:40, goes to the youngest participant in the sample, a 16-year-old student who says she times pees with her friends. The high in the men's category, 2:25 of continuous urine at the middle urinal in the men's room of Yoshi's, an Oakland nightclub, immediately following a performance by Astrud Gilberto on March 4th, 1990, belongs to the author. (For comparison, the longest continuous micturition I have heard of is four minutes, by Griff Kundahl, at Trinka's in Washington, D.C. Kundahl intentionally restricted the flow, however, which disqualifies him.)

Other outstanding showings are 2:10, from a 24-year-old male architecture student, and two minutes from three people: a 37-year-old male professor (without beer), a 29-year-old male attorney, and an 18-year-old female who doesn't give her occupation. 7% of respondents claim they've broken one minute without having consumed beer.

A couple of respondents remark that they achieve their best times upon waking. A graduate student who times his pees "all the time" writes, "usually, if I save up overnight I can break a minute in the morning." Others cite unusual circumstances, like the 27-year-old businessman who recounts, "Once, as a young adolescent, I attended a funeral and was occupied all day. I pulled well, well over a minute."

Natural ability should not be ignored, however. One young man boasts, "I have been complemented on how much my bladder can hold," while another relates, "I've learned that I'm real quick." A teen writes that he has timed his pees, "without really satisfactory results."

A 25-year-old grad student says that his parents got into the act, answering, "I never have, but my parents said they did when I was little, because I would hold it for an unusually long time. They claimed I broke a minute once. Without beer, obviously."

Finally, two more men share stories about related matters. One, a 41-year-old, answers, "No, but I do have a record of sorts. Once on a long bus ride, I had to hold it for about three hours, and it took over five minutes at the next stop to relax enough where I could start peeing. Boy, what a relief!!!" The other, 30, writes, "Never timed, but I have measured volume. Summer of '89 I broke both ankles and spent four days in the hospital. I had to whiz into a jug 'cause I obviously couldn't walk to the restroom. One morning I almost filled the 38 fluid ounce capacity jug."

Do you pee in the shower?

59% say they do, 9% answer that they do it sometimes, and 6% say they do it seldom or occasionally. Meanwhile, only 16% say they don't at all.

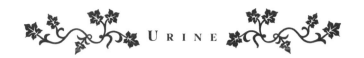

The practice comes highly recommended. Some respondents assert that something about the shower itself makes a body want to pee. One writes, "Oh yeah. It's my favorite place. All that liquid makes you have to *go*!" A 25-year-old propounds, "What better place? The warm rushing water is a natural diuretic."

Others praise the activity's ecological soundness, with the assertions, "It saves a toilet flush worth of H_2O" and "It saves water." A 38-year-old woman relates that in the shower she pees for distance. Another woman writes, "I heard it's good for athlete's foot."

But the most fanatical devotee, a balding, suburban 30-year-old, gives no rationale, seeming instead to be compelled by mysterious inner drives. He answers, "At every possible opportunity. I also pee in sinks and basement floor drains. I used to pee in ashtrays located near urinals when I was in college."

Opponents of in-shower urination would undoubtedly be appalled at the practice's popularity. Their views, expressed well by two teenage respondents who answer, "No, actually it disgusts me that others do," and "Something about peeing in the shower disgusts me," clearly lie in the minority.

(Guys:) Ever pee out the window of a moving car? (Gals:) Ever accidentally pee a little from laughing too much?

I aimed the pee-from-laughing question toward women because I'd heard and read of the phenomenon as being particularly female, but four of the 34 who answered Yes to this question are men responding to the question despite its wording. Similarly, while no woman says she has urinated from a moving car, one tells about her peeing from a bedroom window. In both cases, I probably would have gotten more material had I left the gender specifiers off.

14% of male respondents say they've peed out the window of a moving car. Another says he's done it from a van, and another answers, "Not a moving one." A 47-year-old boasts that the car was going 70 mph.

Six male respondents demonstrate men's propensity to interpret language in competitive terms by answering with, "No, but . . . " These status-maintaining responses are: "No, but I've peed off a bridge onto a convertible Rabbit with the top down and about half of it bounced off the rail and hit me in the leg," "No, but I peed into a plastic bag while driving cross country," "No, but I've peed in a cup whilst driving a car across Kansas in the middle of the night," "No, but peed on myself once on the Jersey Turnpike while on motorcycle," "No, but peed out of dorm window in college," and, perhaps most revealingly, "No, but I have intentionally thrown a bowling ball down the lane when the gate was down."

Among female respondents, 75% say they have experienced "giggle incontinence" (the medical term). One who has not, a 28-year-old who feels that bodily functions are "important to maintain high quality of life," asserts, "No, I have good bladder control." An 18-year-old with her whole life ahead of her replies, "No! Not yet." Two participants say they themselves haven't peed from laughing, but they know people who do. Another says she hasn't done it since she was a kid. Meanwhile, a 21-year-old says it's happened to her "many times." Finally a 20-year-old responds, "Yes. This questionnaire is putting me in a compromising position . . . ."

Ever pee while in a swimming pool? Public or private? Was this recent? How about a hot tub? No way!

Most people in the sample, 67%, say they have added pee to a pool at some point, but most of them, 46% of the total sample, say the contributions were not recent. One 25-year-old punster explains that he only did it as a "wee lad." 7% admit to having done it recently. Some seem abashed, like the young man who answers, "Yes, public, quite recently. I felt bad about it, though." For others, like the 41-year-old who replies, "Sure (slowly)," the practice seems to be standard procedure. 2% even answer that they do it often.

Refuge from another's urine can't be reliably found in private pools, either. More respondents,

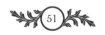

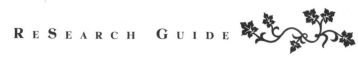

42%, say they urinated in public pools, but a good 30% answer that they've done it in private ones.

5% add that they've peed in the ocean. A woman mentions having urinated in a lake, and a young man says he tinkled in the bathtub when he was little. Another young man tells, "I remember once I was dripping wet and my sister was drying me and I thought I could pee and she wouldn't know; she did."

5% say they have urinated in a hot tub, and another 2% say they're not sure. The real surprise answer, however, comes from a malicious 18-year-old who answers, "Hot tubs, as long as I'm not going to be sitting in it myself."

(Gals:) Ever use the men's room because the line was too long for the women's and it was an "emergency"? (Guys:) Ever find it hard to pee if there's a long line of people waiting behind you? Ever use a toilet stall purely for privacy's sake?

The potty parity problem is so prevalent that 70% of women respondents answer that they have used the men's room for "emergencies." One teen answers, "Yes—and for other reasons." Another writes, "No, I just do it for fun."

A 28-year-old notes, "There is *never* a line at the men's room." A 31-year-old remarks, "Sure, did it today! I've been having bladder infections and you're not supposed to hold it in." Meanwhile, a 28-year-old male respondent reports, "I know of a woman who was arrested for this."

Several men offer names they use for the psychophysical phenomenon described in the first "Guy" question, including "can fright" and "piss shyness." A 37-year-old professor instructs, "This is 'pee shyness.' Happens to some in football stadium pee troughs." 38% of the men report having had this affliction.

One young man remarks that he's especially susceptible to can fright if friends of his are waiting. Another tells of a piss-shy friend of his who had to take a drug test for an employer. Someone had to actually watch him urinate, and as a result, the process took "hours."

As for using a stall for urination privacy, 44% of men say they've done it. An architect says he "will choose stall every time over 'trough' urinals." A grad student says he sometimes uses a stall because he likes to urinate while seated. A programmer mentions that when he's peeing in a toilet stall, he tries to "make as much noise as possible," presumably to discourage interruption.

Do you sometimes briefly shiver in the middle of a long pee?

49% of respondents, mostly men, say they do experience "piss shiver," while 29%, mostly women, say they do not. Comments from Yes-respondents include, "Yes—oh the relief," "With joy, yes," "I'm sorry to admit, yes," and "Yeah, and I can't figure out why."

4% say that piss-shivering happens only when they're cold, 2% say it happens near the end of their urine streams and not in the middle, 4% answer that they don't know if they get it or not, and 1% say it used to happen to them but doesn't anymore. As an aside, a woman shares, "In stressful situations . . . to start to pee I have to tickle a certain spot on my butt."

(Guys:) How do you pee with an early morning erection? Or do you just wait?

26% of the men say they do just wait, making it the most popular solution by far. "Otherwise it's yoga time," explains one. Next, with 11%, comes bending over or leaning forward. A woman answering the question writes, "My boyfriend leans against the wall." A 27-year-old recommends, "Move your butt up in relation to your woody, move back, and judge the angle. I'm good at this." Finally, a 29-year-old relates, "Usually I bend forward and bend my dick, or I think about trees blowing in the wind or grey buildings."

Another 11%, possibly with lower-than-average standing erection angles, say they have no problem or that they just do it. One student answers, "Just aim and go. (My erection goes out, not up)"

8% say they sit down on the toilet. 3% each answer that they try to relax, stand back further, use the shower, or masturbate. A 22-year-old says

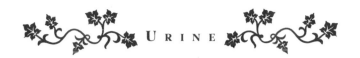
he leans over the bowl while kneeling down. A 30-year-old gives a cryptic response: "Cold water does the trick." A 25-year-old student answers, "I sometimes just let it arc into the bathtub or wait until I'm in the shower. There is something rather satisfying about peeing with a hard-on. Kind of a free feeling."

Where do you like to pee outdoors? Have you ever peed from the top of a tree? Off a cliff?

Respondents like to urinate into bushes and plants or under trees best, with answers in this category accounting for 31% of the sample. One young man warns, however, "Not on the stump of a big tree so it dribbles back downhill at me." 5%, mostly men, say they like to urinate anywhere, everywhere, or in lots of places. Meanwhile another 5%, mostly women, say they don't particularly enjoy alfresco urination. A 30-year-old female archaeologist points out, however, that "in field work you have to go outside." 5% say they just look for someplace private or secluded.

4%, all guys, mention snow. Another 4%, also all men, mention loose soil, dirt, sand, or gravel. A 24-year-old recommends "loose soil that kind of bubbles up."

3%, two women and one man, favor peeing on or in grass, but one 18-year-old woman relates, "grass is last resort." 2% say they like to pee outdoors at night.

Women respondents mention preferring to urinate behind cars or car doors, behind rocks, in doorways, and behind horses. Some women, meanwhile, show a taste for drama. One 23-year-old answers, "someplace secluded and on a hill." A 20-year-old writes, "I like to pee near the ocean on the rocks."

Men mention peeing into streams, onto fences, into holes they've dug, out high windows, into leaves, onto walls in alleys, behind 7-11s or gas stations, and onto compost heaps. One says he likes to pee off the roof of a friend's apartment building. A grad student relates, "I'm told peeing onto an electric fence can be exciting."

A 30-year-old man recalls, "When I was 16 or 17, I kept laying chickens. I was in the habit of pissing on one particular board in the barn near the water faucet." (Gerund adjective "laying," not verb.)

In the follow-up question, only 6% say they have peed from a treetop, and 16%, all men, say they've peed off cliffs. One young woman says she peed off a tree when she was little. Meanwhile, a young man who probably views himself as especially literate writes, "I've done it off a cliff. I thought of the Brontë sisters whilst it." Finally, another young man answers that he has urinated off a cliff "only in dream."

(Guys:) Do you use the fly on underwear, do you pull them down, or do you pull one of the leg holes up and around? Do you favor boxers or briefs?

Flies are unpopular. Only 18% of male respondents say they use the fly on their underwear. As one 20-year-old student puts it, "No male ever uses that fly thing!!!" The most popular method, with 35%, is just to pull the garment down. 9% say they use one of the leg holes.

18% of male participants say they favor boxers, 42% say they favor briefs, 6% say they use both, and 2% say they prefer no undies at all. Preferred undergarment type does not strongly correlate with penis exposure technique; the fly, leg-hole, and waistband groups all show similar brief-to-boxer ratios.

A number of respondents say they usually try to use the fly, but under duress revert to pulling them down, which they consider easier. 17% say they vary their method depending on what type of undies they're wearing, if they're wearing shorts, if the pants have a fly, or even, "urgency of need." A 24-year-old sports promoter answers, "Sometimes. Sometimes. Both. I'm extremely flexible."

(Guys:) Do you usually flush urinals? If not, why not?

This question only appeared on the last version of the questionnaire, and so it was only asked of 24 male participants. Of these, 13 (54%) say they do flush and 8 (33%) say they don't. One

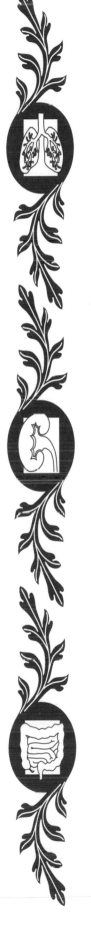

(4%) answers "sometimes." Seven of the eight who don't flush say it's to conserve water. The other one of the eight explains, "Who knows what's on handle?" Some urinal flushers explain that they do it out of habit or because "it stinks." Finally, one young man asks, "What about all the people I see flushing *first*?"

Urine Therapy

In India, Germany, South America, and elsewhere today, millions swear by the health benefits of urine as a salve, a lotion, an eyewash, and a tonic. The practice of drinking a glass of one's own urine each morning, one part of Urine Therapy, came to international attention in the late 1970's with India's Prime Minister Morarji Desai, who advocated the practice in the book *Nature Cure* and kept it in his own routine wherever he went. Octogenarian Desai's excellent health and alertness, against the backdrop of India's folk medicine tradition of urine drinking, lent credibility to his endorsement.

The tradition is documented in sacred Hindu writings such as the *Hathyoga-pradipka* and the *Damar Tantra*, which recommend urine drinking, referring to urine as "shivambu," the water of the Shiva and the water of well-being. It's no coincidence that the practice arose within Hinduism; doctors today know that the toxicity level of a person's urine correlates with how much meat they eat and how much aerobic exercise they get. Because many yogis are sedentary and eat no meat, their urine is almost completely free of toxins, and Hindu writings commend these practices. The "Shivambukalpa," part of the *Damar Tantra*, recommends, "Non-eater of saltish, bitter, and sharp foods, eater of easily digestible and divine foods, free from exertion, controller of the senses . . . the discriminating and high-aiming devotee should urinate facing East. Leaving aside the first and last stream, he should drink the middle stream . . . . Shivambu is a heavenly nectar. It is the destroyer of old age and disease."

Some modern discussions of Urine Therapy include even bolder assertions. The back cover of Dr. C. P. Mithal's 1978 book *Urine Therapy* exclaims, "Free treatment for every man, woman and child! All diseases are curable! No doctor is required! How? Urine Therapy is the answer!" Mithal claims that lost sailors have always enjoyed healthful results from drinking their own urine, and that urine "is a living liquid and specifically made for us by our body. Nothing can be more suitable for our health than our urine." Most of Mithal's book consists of triumphant case histories of Urine Therapy's curing a variety of diseases, but he mentions no controlled studies or cases in which the therapy *failed* to cure the patient.

Mithal also discusses an earlier book by Englishman John W. Armstrong, *The Water of Life*, written after the author felt he had cured himself of tuberculosis and diabetes through a strict regimen of urine drinking and bathing. Armstrong's inspiration came from his own unique interpretation of Proverbs 5:15, which commands, "Drink waters out of thine own cistern," an interpretation which may have come from similar advice in Second Kings 18:31 and Isaiah 36:16, which follow references to eating dung and drinking urine.

While few health professionals would agree with Mithal and Armstrong's broader claims, it is true that urine is a pretty good thing to wash wounds with. In fact, medical history records a case in which a surgeon attended a duel, and when a participant's nose was cut off, the surgeon picked it up and peed on it to clean it. When he stitched it back on shortly afterward, it stayed on. For most people, drinking a little of their own urine every morning, if it makes them feel better, certainly couldn't hurt. Urine actually contains many key nutrients, and, as discussed in the October 1880 *The Lancet*, its chemistry closely resembles that of beef tea, a bouillon-like drink typically made for invalids. The only major difference is that urine contains more urea and uric acid.

Actual Urine Therapy procedures vary, but the one constant is that you always use your own urine. You treat skin problems, wounds, and some

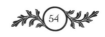

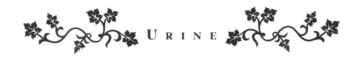

less serious ailments with urine skin packs and washes, using either fresh or week-old urine depending on the condition. Nosebleeds and sinus trouble are treated with "Mutra-Neti," or drawing urine up into the nostrils. For serious diseases, you anoint yourself with urine and then fast on urine and water, recycling your urine through your body repeatedly for days. During this most extreme method of treatment, the rationale goes, all the poisons in your body come out through vomiting, diarrhea, and skin eruptions, leaving you purified and cured.

Many cultures also drink urine not for health but for ceremonial greeting and toasting rituals.

Prince Albert in a Can: Urination Experiences with Genital Piercings

People's urinary habits are affected by genital piercings such as the Prince Albert, in which a ring enters a man's urethra and exits underneath at the base of his glans. As sexy as many find the Prince Albert (hereafter, PA), it does come at the price of urinary convenience. Exiting urine adheres to the ring, following it around and causing a spray. When the ring is out, the urine sprays or forms two streams, one at each end of the pierce. The added urine pathway can also mean an increase in terminal dribbling. To find out more about people's experiences with piercings and urination, I posted a query to the Internet newsgroup *rec.arts.bodyart*. Seventeen people responded, providing the following information:

At urinals, men with PA's usually twist the ends of their penises up so the underside faces the wall. A few take a different angle, turning the penis upside-down. One man explains, "I found that if I just grab the loose skin on the top of the shaft, just below the head, and flip the whole proposition over, the multiple streams will all arch into the urinal instead of down my pants leg." A man with eight rings in his PA describes another strategy: "Standing at the urinal, not vertically, but with my feet

planted in the customary position and my head resting against the wall over the urinal usually reduces the back-splash." Another man explains, "[When I'm not wearing my ring] I use my index finger to cover the hole with a slight amount of pressure and just piss normally."

Everyone agrees that the most reliable method, however, is to sit on a toilet. One man adds that, "Having a PA will definitely make you sympathize with women about leaving the toilet seat down . . . . It only took me one trip straight to the bottom of the bowl, arse first, to learn that lesson. Furthermore, I believe that my thighs have definitely shaped up a bit from squatting inches above public toilets when no urinal is available." But another man notes that peeing sitting down causes more dribbling afterwards than using a urinal does.

Another solution comes from the man who explains, "[I] have a hospital urinal next to my bed; I can fit the entire head of my dick into it, and nothing goes astray." A couple of people pointed out that thicker jewelry makes changing urinary habits more necessary. One man explains, "My PA is a 2 gauge and I am definitely a setter and not a pointer anymore."

Although most of the Internet respondents wrote specifically about urinating with a PA, a few touched on other issues. One woman writes, "after I got my labia pierce, urinating stung horribly for about 10 days . . . .[Now I] have to dab *very* carefully with toilet paper." Finally, a young man shares, "My new PA does add a new twist to the act of urination, but having just observed a post-PA orgasm for the first time, I'll tell ya, PA cumming is a whole lot more interesting than PA peeing. I was lying down and anticipating being drenched from the neck down, but now it flies straight up in the air and lands in one big glob on my stomach. It sent me into hysterics."

All About Urine

From the biological (and topological) perspective, vertebrates are shaped like donuts or tubes.

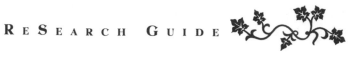

We have one big hole going through us, our digestive tract. In this description, the tract's contents lie outside the body, and its lining is a specialized exterior surface devoted to digestion and excretion just as our skin is an exterior surface devoted primarily to sensation, protection, and temperature control. The undigestible portion of what you eat, the fiber, etc, never actually enters your body; it just travels next to this interior surface for a day or so.

Urine is a different story. Ingested liquids do not simply pass through you, undigested or not, and become urine. All of your urine was genuinely inside of your body, in your blood stream. Your heart pumped it around, along with the rest of your blood, your kidneys decided you didn't need it (to ascribe intention) and filtered it out, it collected in your bladder, and you excreted it. Urine travels a long and complicated route, and beer urine is no exception.

Adults normally void their urine five to seven times per day, producing a total of one to one-and-a-half liters. Age and sex do not appreciably influence this amount, but the season does; we urinate more during winter. And, of course, drinking more increases the amount, while sweating more, or bleeding profusely, decreases it. Gravity affects this balance; in zero gravity, astronauts want to urinate more and drink less, because their body fluids drift up and give the brain faulty signals. Men typically urinate for 15 to 20 seconds; however, one study found that in "military situations," the average male urine duration was 45 seconds.

Adult men's urine streams are usually narrower than adult women's, because sexual experience and childbirth can alter a woman's labial tissues and make her urine stream more fanlike or ribbonlike. An old test of maidenhood exploited this connection: if a young woman could produce a urine stream like a man's, it argued that she was a virgin.

Urine's normal yellow color comes from urochrome, a yellow pigment produced from the breakdown of hemoglobin. Urine sometimes becomes cloudy during the summer when alkaline salts in fruit cause phosphates to precipitate out of it, or in winter, when uric acid or urates precipitate out. Large doses of Riboflavin (Vitamin B_2) color it bright yellow, while consuming methylene blue or indigo dye will make it blue-green. Taking L-Dopa turns it dark brown. Eating rhubarb, senna (a purgative herb), or cascara (a laxative tree bark) can turn acidic urine brownish and alkaline urine pinkish. Santonin, in wormwood, can also turn alkaline urine pink. Some people have a genetic trait that causes beets to redden their urine as well.

Another trait gives some people's urine a characteristic smell after they eat asparagus. Drinking turpentine, meanwhile, imparts a rose-like scent to the urine, and some high-born Roman ladies perfumed their urine in this way, despite turpentine's poison, accepting a similar trade-off to the one presented by another practice of that class, eating the deadly nightshade to acquire the alluringly dilated pupils expected of a *bella donna*.

The kidneys produce urine constantly, even when the bladder is full. When the bladder reaches capacity during the night, it results in nocturia, the need to get up and pee. Most people experience nocturia episodically, after drinking a lot of fluids, and older people experience it regularly, rising once per night for every decade of age over 50, on the average.

Incontinence, involuntary urination, may result from a too-full bladder, but other causes, such as extreme fright, may trigger it as well. "Giggle incontinence," as the medical literature calls it, is another form of incontinence resulting from intense laughter. It occurs most often in adolescent girls, and has affected one-quarter of the population at least once. Some women also experience occasional incontinence during sexual intercourse. In the discussion that their textbook *Urodynamics, Principles, Practice, and Application* (1984) gives to this topic, Mundy, Stephenson and Wein point out that, "Although the widely read devotee of 'men's' magazines may regard it [incontinence during coitus] as almost fashionable, most patients and their partners find it upsetting." Intense involvement in other activities

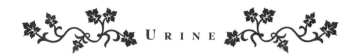

can also lead to incontinence, although you might debate in these cases whether or not the urination is truly involuntary. In Las Vegas, for example, security guards have had to drag away slot machine players who wouldn't quit playing for long enough to visit the bathroom.

Men, meanwhile, frequently contend with "terminal dribbling," the medical name for the phenomenon described by the familiar graffito, "No matter how you shake and dance/The last drops always go down your pants" (variation: ". . .pull and squeeze/. . .down your knees").

Ideally, the urine leaves the body completely, but sometimes a residue builds up in its path, producing stones in the kidneys or the bladder. Large stones can cause pain and require surgical removal. Stones vary in composition, but nearly always contain as main ingredients calcium oxalate (which is also the main ingredient in dental calculus), uric acid, and calcium phosphate.

Men are more likely to form kidney stones than women, and for people who do form them, production typically peaks at around age 50. Kidney stone formation correlates with intake of animal protein, and vegetarians rarely get stones. For this reason, the percentage of people in this country who get kidney stones has increased over the century, the average age at which they first show up has decreased, and their occurrence has correlated with affluence.

Bladder stones, on the other hand, are rare in industrialized countries and occur more frequently in children of the third world whose diets consist primarily of polished rice. Bladder stones can reach 8 cm in diameter and when sliced in half reveal a beautiful, geode-like layering pattern.

Because urine carries the by-products of much of the body's chemical activities, including metabolizations and phagocytosis, chemical analysis of the urine, urinalysis, can provide a detailed log of what a person has ingested and been exposed to. Hence the now-nearly-standard workplace urine test.

The amount of "clean" time required beforehand for a drug test to yield a negative result var-

ies widely. The body stores away traces of some drugs, so for these, two numbers apply, one for the occasional user and one for the habitué. Examples of these are marijuana (up to three days occasional/up to six weeks habitual), barbiturates (up to three days/one month), and Benziodiazepines, such as Valium and Librium (can show up in ex-frequent users for months afterwards).

The traces of other drugs, however, vacate the body more rapidly. Such drugs include cocaine, amphetamines, opiates, and LSD, which can take up to two or three days, and PCP, which can take up to a week (and for which Thorazine and other drugs can give false positives). Until recently, eating poppy seeds could give a false positive for opiates up to 60 hours after ingestion, but it has been found that analysis for 6-O-acetylmorphine, a metabolite of heroin, can distinguish heroin use in opiate positive urine.

Naturally, some ne'er-do-wells have come up with ways of defeating urine tests, or at least increasing the likelihood of their coming out negative. Some of the methods listed by the National Institute on Drug Abuse, a part of the U.S. Department of Health and Human Services, in one of their publications, include putting chemicals under the fingernails and releasing them into the specimen, drinking lots of water for several hours before the test, poking a small hole in the bottom of the specimen container so all the urine leaks out during shipping, and adding salt, detergent, dispenser soap, tap water, or other convenient adulterants. They recommend the counter-measures of watching the actual voiding of the urine, or at least measuring its temperature immediately afterwards.

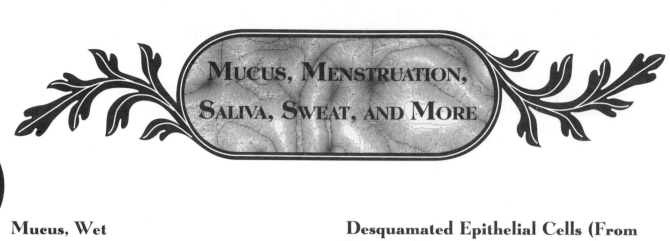
Mucus, Wet

SNOT, GUBBINS, PHLEGM, LOOGIE, GOB, HAWKER, GILBERT, SPUTUM

Mucus, Dried

NOSEPICK, BOOGERS, BOOGIES, TEPHRA, SLEEP-ERS, SLEEP, EYE BOOGERS, GREEBLIES

Saliva/To Spill Saliva

SPIT, SPITTLE, SLOBBER, SLAVER, DRIVEL, DROOL

To (Clear Your Throat And) Spit

EXPECTORATE, HAWK A LOOGIE, HORK A GOB, GOB

Menstrual Fluid

MENSTRUAL BLOOD, CATAMENIAL FLUID

Menstruation

MENSES, MONTHLIES, PROBLEM DAYS, COURSES, THAT TIME, PERIOD, THE CURSE, OLD FAITHFUL

I'm Menstruating

I'M ILL/INDISPOSED/IN USE/UNDER THE WEATHER/ UNAVAILABLE, IT'S MY TIME OF THE MONTH, I'M ON THE RAG, THE CARDINAL IS AT HOME, MY CHERRY'S IN SHERRY (BEAT SLANG), I'M A COMMUNIST (BEAT SLANG), I HAVE A VISITOR, A FRIEND, AUNT FLO, THE PAINTERS IN, THE RED KING (GERMANY), JACQUES/FRANÇOIS/MARTIN (FRANCE), FREDERICK BARBAROSSA (GERMANY; BARBAROSSA WAS "RED BEARD"), I FELL OFF THE ROOF (SOUTHERN)

Semen

JIZ, JAZZ, LIQUOR OF LOVE, CUM, CUM SHOT, SPERM, SPEW, WAD, LOAD, CREAM, JERK JUICE, JOY JUICE, JUNK, GUNK, SCUM, SCUZZ, SPUNK, MILT

Desquamated Epithelial Cells (From Various Regions)

SMEGMA, TOE CHEESE, TOE JAM, DANDRUFF, BELLY BUTTON LINT

Phlegm, mucus, semen, saliva, sweat, earwax, belly button lint, and other minor players in the bodily functions game don't have vast cultural and intellectual traditions behind them like big guns such as feces do, but they nevertheless each have special strengths of their own. Loose mucus and the dried mucus-impurity conglomerates we call "boogers" pose problems in the area of etiquette. Our unique sweat sets us apart from other mammals, while vestiges of our more scent-oriented evolutionary past make sweat and vaginal secretions key ingredients in the mystery of romance. Semen, earwax, smegma, sebum, tears, and other excretions, meanwhile, each have short stories of their own.

Menstruation, meanwhile, is no minor player, having greatly influenced many elements of culture, particularly religion, social tradition, social structure, folklore, politics, and even agriculture. This book de-emphasizes reproduction, so it shortchanges menstruation, but the one chapter that covers it should provide a glimpse of some of the larger areas in which the function has played an important role.

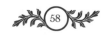

People, Places, and Picking (Survey)

Nasal Hygiene Section

Where, typically, do you pick your nose (bathroom, car, kitchen. . .)?

Fortunately, only one person, a 22-year-old woman who writes that she "revels" in bodily functions, mentions "kitchen" as one of her favorite hunting grounds. The rest of us favor, in descending order, the bathroom, the car, the bedroom, bed itself, our homes, our desks at work, the living room, the shower, in front of the television, and on public transportation, the library, outside, the elevator, and on bicycle. 18% answer that they'll pick anywhere at all, 10% say they'll do it anywhere they have privacy, and a thrill-seeking 4% do it anywhere they feel no one is looking. Women and men tend to pick different places. Women more often favor bedrooms and bathrooms, while men are more likely to pick in cars or anywhere at all.

Several respondents say they pick their noses in bed before going to sleep, and one undoubtedly large-boogered woman explains that she has trouble breathing if she doesn't. A polite but troubled 26-year-old man who seeks privacy when picking writes, "Sometimes, in the presence of others, the feeling in my nose makes me wonder whether I have picked in public." A 35-year-old male musician explains that he picks his nose "when pretty girls aren't looking." Meanwhile, with refreshingly pure consumerist zeal, a mother of two writes, "I pick my nose in the bathroom — my brand of toilet paper is softer than most Kleenex."

4% of the sample claim they don't pick their noses at all.

What do you do with the "boogers" once you've snagged them?

34% flick, drop, or toss them away. A good portion of this predominately male group mention rolling them first, usually between the fingers or on pants. Some booger flickers make sport with their tiny projectiles: a 19-year-old woman answers, "Flick them at my roommate," a 20-year-old-man explains, "Flick them across the room and see if I can hear them land," and a 36-year-old "dyke artist" writes, "Fling them out the window at traffic lights."

30% wipe them in various places. Wipers like furniture best, with 9% of respondents wiping on, underneath, or onto the undersides of furniture. Other destinations mentioned, in descending order of popularity, are any inconspicuous places, car carpets, bottoms of shoes, carpets, walls behind furniture, pockets, pants, the ground, and boyfriends.

26% put the booger in some form of paper and throw it in the garbage or flush it away. This is the most popular method among women, whose bathroom and bedroom picking habits bring them closer to sources of tissue. Meanwhile, 12% say they throw away or flush but make no mention of paper. Combining these two groups makes throwing away or flushing nose litter, with or without paper, the most popular option.

The dark horse is, of course, eating. 10% say they eat their boogers, and as the stereotype would dictate, this group contains super-proportional numbers of male computer professionals and computer science students. One male student on the Internet answers, "Eat them unless there are too many nasal hairs mixed in." A male software engineer explains, "I usually chuck them. . .though I admit to occasionally scarfing a particularly tasty-looking one." 3% write that they wash the boogers down the drain. Meanwhile, a 31-year-old student writes, "Flick them on the ground. If they are sticky I lick them off and then spit them on the ground."

Ever give yourself a nosebleed from excessively vigorous picking?

61% say this never happened to them and 31% say it has, many adding that it happened a long time ago. Neither group likes the prospect. "Yuck,

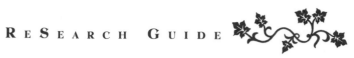

no" and "Never—that's really pathological!" come from the No group, while the Yes people answer with remarks such as "Yeah. Once. Don't recommend it," and "Yes, is there treatment for me?" The only possibly hopeful response comes from a teen who writes "Not yet."

Two No people mention that they have, however, picked bloody boogers, and one Yes carefully qualifies his response with "Only if I already had a nosebleed and picked the scab. (Nosebleed originally not caused by picking)."

6% say they weren't sure or couldn't recall. One of these says it might have happened when it was "really dry out."

Finally, one 20-year-old jokester asks, "Isn't that the goal?"

Would you say you "enjoy" picking your nose?

Respondents divide into four camps on this one: Yes (39%), No (36%), Like The Results (13%), and Sometimes (12%).

In the Yes category, a 31-year-old "baker, student, and fine artist" writes, "Yes, it is very gratifying, an achievement, fulfilling!" and a 22-year-old import purchase agent writes, "I love it. It's cleansing, refreshing."

The No respondents typically stay more down to earth. As one student puts it, "It's a job, not an adventure." Another student writes that she wishes she didn't have to because, "I don't want to stretch my nostrils."

The Like The Results people talk of being able to breathe, feeling good afterwards, and the satisfying feeling of accomplishment, but they all make it clear that the nose-picking act itself gives them no pleasure. Several Sometimes people, on the other hand, enjoy a big catch. One answers, "Yes, if the booger is long enough." Another writes, "Only if I get the big booger I'm after."

The most evocative Sometimes response, however, comes from a 26-year-old man who explains, "It's nothing I get overly excited about, except occasionally."

If so, do you ever do anything to ensure that there'll be plenty to pick (hike dusty trails, snort bread-crumbs...)?

Only 6% answer Yes to this, mentioning volunteering to clean the chalkboards, going on bicycle rides, living in LA, and sniffing cocaine. Meanwhile, several No respondents mention activities they enjoy primarily for other reasons which sow good boogers as well. A middle-aged software developer answers, "Not deliberately, but the old woodworking shop does provide good starter." An architecture student writes, "No, but it was sort of fun to live in NYC because the pickings got all black from soot." A 30-year-old "student-archaeologist" shares that "working as an archaeologist does tend to produce mucus." Finally, a waiter describes, "I once made a booger board for people at a camp I worked at where the mountain dust made for sweet boogies. It was a display case, really."

Finally, a 21-year-old male graduate student in Computer Science gives an effective, all-natural solution: "Sometimes I save up a big snot rather than pick it, for a satisfying session of nose-picking later."

Ever picked anyone else's nose? Whose? How old were you?

75% answer that they never have, with attitudes ranging from "No! I only pick mine!" and "No! (oooh gross)" to a more liberal "No, never. I would, though." One teenager takes the opportunity to repeat the familiar playground proverb, "You can pick your friends [and] you can pick your nose, but you can't pick your friend's nose."

11% say they have picked the noses of others, including family members, boyfriends and girlfriends, and dogs. An 18-year-old answers, "Various boyfriends, any age. You're never too old to pick others' noses." Another young woman coyly answers, "No, but I have a friend who can't resist my nose." A young man relates, "Yes. I performed booger transplants in high school bio class."

Ever place objects in your nostrils (coins, marbles. . .)? Ever "lose" anything up there? How did you finally get it out (if you ever did, that is)?

61% answer No and 18% answer that they've placed objects there but never lost them. Insertables mentioned include rings, pens, pencils, marbles, peanuts, coins, paper wads, beans,

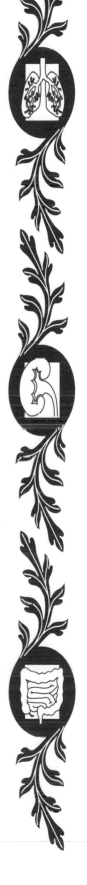

M&Ms, straws, and pen caps.

A 22-year-old woman answers, "No, but my mom always warned me about it." Several respondents tell of nasally incorporating beans and other small objects as children and being taken to tweezer-wielding grandparents or emergency rooms as a result. A 25-year-old recounts, "Sister did—a washer—it was never found." One 28-year-old woman recalls how a boy named Bill Baum from kindergarten put a green pencil eraser up there and started showing it off as a giant booger, but that he soon lost it up there and cried until the teacher made him blow it out. A young man who describes himself as having a weird sense of humor answers, "When I was five I stuck lima beans up my nose. Now I'm a bit more mature and stick to pencils, pens, and straws." Other writing implement enthusiasts include a 25-year-old grad student ("Maybe pencils for a walrus impersonation, but nothing else.") and a 37-year-old Geology professor ("Pencils to make me sneeze. Try it!").

Perhaps the strangest answer comes from a 25-year-old who attributes his love of putting objects into his nose and the feeling of security it provides him with to the first few days of his life, during which he, as a premature infant in an incubator, had no physical contact with people but did have oxygen tubes up his nostrils.

Did you ever deposit a booger someplace you wish you hadn't? Where might that have been?

Most people, 57%, say they have not. A young man who says he's a "fan" of bodily functions responds, "Never. I've always felt fine wherever I leave 'em (my parents, however, would beg to differ, I'm sure)."

About a third of the booger-placement regrets involve furniture and books. Respondents specifically mention undersides of desks and tables, bedside dressers, sofas, and library books. One man regrets his mucous pollution of a book he loaned to a young woman; another mentions having wiped one on furniture at his girlfriend's house. As one young woman points out, it's "not quite a friendly gesture, ya know?"

A male grad student recalls flipping an especially large booger into the air while watching television and hearing it hit somewhere but not knowing where. "Some time later," he explains, "a friend of mine found it pasted on a map hanging on the wall. I denied knowing what it was or how it got there."

Other regretted booger depositories mentioned include a shirt, a bed, a wall, a door, someone's food, an elevator's hand grips, the window of the family camper, and, mentioned by a civic cleanliness-minded 28-year-old, "on the street."

Do you like the actor Slim Pickens?

I included this question as a possibly amusing throwaway figuring that most of us probably admired Mr. Pickens's work and enjoyed his name. I was wrong. 42% indicate that they don't know him or have never heard of him, and many of those who do apparently know of him dislike him.

Some of those who like Mr. Pickens praise him for specific screen accomplishments, such as *Dr. Strangelove* and *The Flim-Flam Man*. Others admire aspects of his persona, such as his "kinda cool" look and his voice.

Slim's detractors aren't generally so specific, as exemplified by the 19-year-old who answers in the largest, darkest letters on the page, "NO!" An exception is the 30-year-old Denver resident who writes, "Not just no, but Hell No. He's possibly one of the very worst 'actors' that hit the big time. I mean, name a flick other than *Dr. Strangelove* that had 'Slim' in it and didn't suck for air. In fact, I use him as a leading indicator for bad flicks."

Do you blow your nose? What are some unusual things you've blown your nose into when you haven't had a tissue or hanky?

2% say they don't blow their noses. Others say they only do it occasionally. But for the rest, the world provides a bounty of nose blowing alternatives.

Cloth objects are the most frequently cited handkerchief substitutes, mentioned by a total of 45% of respondents. In descending order of popularity, these are: shirts (often used when already dirty and after exercising), cloth towels, general "laundry,"

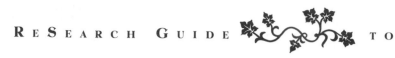

sheets/pillowcases, socks, sweaters/pullovers, ski gloves/mittens, underwear, bathrobes, silk scarves, "roommate's pants cuff," and "some piece of cloth." A towel user writes, "If I have a bad cold I'll usually keep a towel handy by the bedside rather than go through a zillion tissues."

Alternative paper products follow the cloth objects in frequency of mention, receiving 21% of the vote and encompassing paper bags, paper towels, paper napkins, tampon wrappers, newspapers, and magazines. One connoisseur of the press writes, "I've used magazines. Slick paper feels classier, but pulp is satisfying." A woman writes that she uses "scraps of paper (directions, phone numbers) in my glove compartment."

15% say they blow directly into their hands, with some adding that they then wash them in the sink.

11% mention blowing into the air (see next question). A male songwriter-musician answers with, "The air, puking out who knows what through my nose on psychiatric drugs." Meanwhile, a young woman of 22 recalls, "Someone once blew their nose on me—and it was the most awful experience of my life."

8% list leaves and 3% list showers, pools, or Jacuzzis. A young woman mentions having blown into a horse's mane and a 29-year-old attorney says he has blown his nose into a cup. Meanwhile, two respondents mention unusual things they've blown out of their noses: insects and spaghetti.

Finally, a 41-year-old man who describes himself as a "supermasochist" answers, "Sheree's blouse."

Ever blow your nose into "thin air"? Where did it land? Ever blow your nose in the shower?

Most men indicate that they've noseblown into the air, while most women say they have not. Further confirming the gender bias, a male student answers, "Totally, but only with other males." Meanwhile, 40%, with no strong gender correlation, say they've noseblown in the shower.

Like Slim Pickens, nose blowing into thin air, also called "farmer's blow," "Farmer Johns,"

"snarking," "nature blow," "air blow" and "farmer's hankie," causes disagreement. Defenders include a carpenter who brags, "I can spit with my nose in the morning" and a student who explains that he learned the trick from a bicyclist who said it was common practice among serious cyclists but "messy for people riding behind." One admiring observer recalls, "My brother blew one about ten feet and it made a slap sound when it hit the wall."

Opponents, meanwhile, often bring up bad experiences. A driver writes, "Yes, landed on my shirt. Never did it again." A research assistant, seemingly with a fondness for extremely obscure films, answers, "Yes, once after seeing a cultural anthropology film about Middle-Easterners blowing out their nose onto the street. . . [I] felt like I was tearing nasal membranes to 'project' far enough."

Snarkers mention that their mucus landed on the grass, ground, or sidewalk, on their faces, shirts, or shoes, in the trash, on someone's food, and on a sister. Another mentions having once done a farmer's blow off a ski resort chair lift.

While opinions may differ on the nature blow, they're unanimous regarding nose blowing in the shower: it's good. No one disparages the practice, and several recommend it. One young man answers, "In the shower I do everything but defecate." Another writes, "Shower snot attacks are particularly satisfying." Several people say they always blow their noses in the shower, as a part of their routine.

Do you ever sneeze gobs of mucus onto your hand? What do you do with them if you don't have a hanky handy?

75% answer that this has happened to them. The most popular solution, with 17%, is to wipe it onto clothing, specifically pants/jeans, skirts, socks, and the insides of pants pockets. As one 32-year-old writes, "That's what Levi's are for." A seventeen-year-old woman defends, "I wiped it on my skirt! What would you have me do? Eat it?"

12% simply say they wipe it somewhere non-specific. 8% say they wipe it onto the carpet, the

floor, the ground, or the grass. Another 8% go wash their hands, one of them an 18-year-old who gives the panicked answer, "Wash! Excessively." 6% report going and finding a tissue, napkin, or hanky somewhere, including another panicky teen who writes, "Hold my face and run to the nearest tissue."

5% of the sample say they eat it, with two of them adding "of course." Scattered responses of less than 4% each come in for wiping on towels, blankets, shoe soles, grass, backpacks, laundry, trees, buildings, walls, and "some textile." 3% mention rubbing it into hand or arm skin and flicking or flinging it away.

A male of 31 describes his unique solution as, "I slurp them off my hand and spit them on the ground," a similar operation to the one he uses to handle sticky boogers. Finally, an 18-year-old answers, "No, but my sister's nose explodes every time she sneezes and she usually ends up with a handful of snot." Further details are not given.

Miscellaneous Body Products

Mucus

Mucus is flexible stuff. Like Strawberry Jell-O™, mucus is a colloid, which is a tangle of long protein molecules held together with weak bonds and trapping a lot of liquid in between. As a result, mucus can behave as either a liquid or a gel. It traps foreign matter and can act as a conveyor belt to take it away. It binds and transports large quantities of water and solutes. It "coats, soothes, and protects." In addition, mucus contains antiseptic enzymes and immunoglobins, furthering its protective power. With all these features, there's no wonder why, when it comes to secretions, the respiratory, digestive, and reproductive systems rely on mucus.

The lower intestine coats feces with a thin layer of mucus to help it move smoothly, and the cervix and mouth produce mucus for the cleaning and protection they require, but the respiratory system, which takes in an onslaught of irritants, foreign particles, and infectious agents with every breath, puts mucus to its fullest test. A blanket of mucus lines the entire system, from inside the nose and up into the sinuses, Eustachian tubes, and middle ear, down through the throat, and into the bronchial tree and lungs.

As it is secreted, mucus rises out of this mucous membrane, while cilia, microscopic whip-like structures that line much of the system, beat constantly underneath, in waves, propelling the mucous blanket and whatever it contains toward the pharynx, where it is swallowed. Stomach acids then destroy the trapped bacteria. The mucous blanket is renewed through this process about every twenty-five minutes.

In the early 1960's, scientists studying mucous transport performed some revealing experiments that involved depriving chickens of water, to thicken their mucus, and then spreading India ink on their noses. The researchers noted that the ink beneath the surface moved faster than the ink above, suggesting that an inner, more liquid layer of mucus on the chickens' noses drives the movement of the mucous blanket as a whole. Subsequent experiments have confirmed this finding in humans.

In areas with cilia, mucus and deposits move at about 14 millimeters per minute. In unciliated areas, however, such as in the front of the nose, where temperatures fall below the levels cilia can tolerate, progress is much slower. In these areas, the mucous blanket creeps along the surface solely through traction from neighboring, ciliated areas. Fortunately, our nostrils evolved to be of a size that permits our fingers to sidestep this slow process by clearing mucus and deposits from the area directly.

Saliva

The salivary glands produce about half a liter of saliva per day, divided evenly between resting, unstimulated flow and salivation from eating. The resting flow rate during waking hours is about 20 milliliters per hour. During sleep, however, flow slows down dramatically, to about 10 ml.

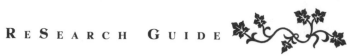
total during eight hours of sleep.

Saliva has many functions. It cleans, lubricates, and prevents drying of the mouth. It dissolves foods and aids in swallowing, and it contains amylase, which begins the digestion of carbohydrates (and which is absent in the saliva of carnivores). Saliva production regulates body water balance by controlling thirst, which comes from the mouth's drying out. Saliva contains blood clotting factors and therefore accelerates blood coagulation, which is a good reason to lick your wounds. The body even uses saliva as a medium to excrete various drugs, metals, and other chemicals.

Not surprisingly, saliva affects dental health, preserving the teeth and protecting them against foreign bacteria. When one produces more saliva, it becomes thinner and contains more calcium—hence, fewer cavities result. People with thicker saliva—saliva with higher viscosity, adhesiveness ("tack"), or a tendency to form strands ("ropiness," "spinnbarkeit," or "Weisenberg effect")—tend to have higher caries rates.

The largest component of dental plaque, which forms out of saliva, is living bacteria. Plaque is a mass of tightly-packed microorganisms participating in a local ecology too closely-interwoven for foreign bacteria to penetrate. We pay a price for their protection, however, because the resident bacteria themselves cause problems, forming cavities and tartar, or calculus, which can lead to cavities.

It is possible to make a mouthwash which completely removes and prevents plaque and is safe for prolonged use, by using the chemical chlorhexidine glucona. The catch is that chlorhexidine glucona mouthwashes also stain the teeth brown and have a lingering unpleasant aftertaste. Meanwhile, commercial mouthwashes do kill millions of germs on contact, as advertised, but they leave billions more of the troublesome but necessary microorganisms unharmed.

Tears and Sleepers

Under normal circumstances, we produce 1.5 microliters of tears per minute, which means that we secrete tears at about the same rate as we manufacture urine. The tear film that covers our eyeballs consists of three layers. The thickest layer, comprising 75% of the volume, is a layer of mucin, from the goblet cells, that lies directly on the surface of the eyeball. On top of this, comprising about 24% of the volume, is an aqueous layer from the lachrymal glands. Separating the aqueous layer from the air is a thin layer of oils, from the Meibomian glands in the eyelids, which prevents the aqueous layer from evaporating.

Along with water, mucin, and lipids, tears contain lysozome (an antibacterial protein), immunoglobins, glucose, urea, sodium, and potassium. Tears function to fill irregularities in the cornea for better optics, kill bacteria, lubricate the eye socket, ball, and lid, and wash away debris and noxious substances, including particles and irritants from the air and dead cells. Like saliva, tears also serve as a medium for the excretion of certain drugs.

In addition to flowing down the cheeks, tears and their debris wash away into is the nose, which connects to the eyes via the nasolachrymal ducts. Each eye has a lower and an upper entrance to these ducts. You can see the lower entrance ("punctum") as a small hole in the inner part of the rim of the lower eyelid. The presence of these ducts explains why crying stuffs up your nose and why some people can blow air bubbles from their eyes underwater, by plugging their noses and slowly "blowing."

Tears are mostly mucin, which solidifies rapidly when removed from the surface of the eyeball. At night, when eyes remain closed for a long time, capillary action can draw away tears pooled in the corner of the eye and move them onto the skin, where they dry out and solidify into "sleepers."

Earwax

Earwax, or cerumen, comes from sebaceous glands and ceruminous glands (which are modified sebaceous glands) that lie just inside the ear. It protects the ear, but has only mild antibacterial properties and, one expert notes, no insect-repellent properties at all.

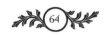

There are two different types of earwax. People of Asian and American descent have dry, scaly earwax, while most descendants of Africans and Europeans have a moister earwax that darkens with exposure to air. In addition, individuals vary widely in the amount of cerumen they produce. Some people churn out enough of it to block their ear canal and require medical attention. Age affects earwax as well. Older people have drier earwax, with less of the sebaceous component." Occasionally one accumulates enough earwax to actually diminish hearing-hence the expression, "Got wax in your ears?"

Smegma, Toe Cheese, Belly button Lint, Dandruff

Body surface odors come from microbial breakdown of sweat, sebum, and scaled-off skin cells. Different bacteria digest these materials into different sets of chemicals. Meanwhile, the mixture of bacteria species varies over different body regions. As a result, the odor-determining chemical mixtures produced on the skin of different parts of the body also vary.

Especially strong scents will come from any moist areas where these desquamated epithelial cells can build up, such as on scalps, under toenails, in navels, and under foreskins. In these places, the bacteria have a feast, generating hefty quantities of the local odorants.

The scalp, for example, is home to the yeast Pityrosporum ovale, which produces gamma-lactones, fruity odorants that characterize scalp odor. Bacteria in the underarm produce sweaty-smelling chemicals such as androstenone and isovaleric acid. Microbes in the navel and penis mix cocktails of their own. The strongest smells, however, come from the foot, where Corynebacteria, close relatives of the Brevibacteria found in dairy products, produce methane thiol, a major component of cheddar cheese aroma. Some feet also harbor Pseudomonas bacteria, which produce odorous sulfur compounds such as dimethyl disulfide (cabbage odor) and methyl

mercaptan (another cheese odor), and Proteus bacteria, which produce sulfur compounds as well as amine compounds (fishy odors).

Substances such as smegma and toe cheese, then, are a mixture of skin secretions and dead cells, along with the bacteria that live off of them and the cheesy, cabbage-y, and fishy-smelling waste products they produce as a result.

Milk

Biologically, milk defines us. We named the taxonomic class we belong to, Mammalia, after the Latin word for breast, *mamma*, because it was milk production, not hair or warm blood or live birth, that granted our early mammalian ancestors more time to develop, opening a new evolutionary branch. To quote the band They Might Be Giants, milk stands in between extinction in the cold and explosive radiating growth.

Because men can make big money selling baby formula, companies such as Nestlé have promoted the idea that breast-feeding is old-fashioned and distasteful, even in countries where preparing formula with available water and storage almost assures death for the infant consumers. In 1981, after years of public outcry, the U.N. reined in the industry by passing the World Health Organization's International Code on Marketing Breast Milk Substitutes, with the United States casting the sole negative ballot among 119 nations. A few years later, however, Surgeon General C. Everett Koop, recognizing breast-feeding's health benefits, held a workshop to encourage the practice in all segments of the country's population. In the meantime, formula manufacturers have been feeling the pinch of an increasingly informed public. In 1971, only one-quarter of the infants in this country were nursed. Now the number exceeds two-thirds.

Milk's whole reason for being is to assure health and growth, so it contains a lot of nutrients and other beneficial components. Along with protein, carbohydrates (mostly lactose), and fat, milk supplies a vitamin-pill-like ingredient list of vitamins, minerals (including 280 milligrams per liter of

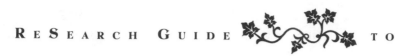

calcium), and trace elements, as well as antibodies built up by the mother (which formula lacks) to bolster the baby's immune system.

During the child's early infancy, mother's milk changes to meet the child's needs. Days one to five produce colostrum, which has less lactose than mature milk and more protein, Vitamin E, Vitamin B_{12}, salt, zinc, and beta-carotene, the last of which gives it a yellowish color. Between days six and eleven, the milk shifts from colostrum over to mature milk, which is bluish. Of all mammal milks, human milk has the lowest concentrations of protein, calcium, and phosphorus and the highest concentration of lactose, matching our relatively slow growth and the high sugar requirements of our brains.

Per liter, mature milk contains about 73 grams of lactose, 9 grams of protein, and 40 grams of fat, totaling about 700 calories, a little over half of which come from the fat. Fat content varies widely, however, from person to person, feeding to feeding, and even within a single feeding; as the baby drinks, the fat content rises.

Along with the nutrients, milk also contains other chemicals from the foods the mother has eaten. Garlic, brussels sprouts, and other foods eaten by the mother can give the infant gas. Coffee can keep it awake. Excessive amounts of alcohol can get it drunk. Ingested foods also alter the milk's flavor, and after weaning, breast-fed babies tend to be more willing to eat unfamiliar foods than babies who were raised on bland, unvarying formula.

Milk production finishes a woman's reproductive cycle. During pregnancy, women gain eight to ten pounds extra, beyond the weight of the fetus, placenta, and fluid, to prepare for lactating, and, reflecting this, women who nurse return to their baseline weights more quickly than those who do not. Delivery of the placenta, which discontinues the presence of placental hormones, triggers lactation initially, and mothers who retain part of the placenta produce no milk until the remaining fragments are removed.

Following birth, the mother will produce milk for as long as the baby continues drinking it. Sucking on the nipple stimulates the release of two hormones, prolactin and oxytocin. Prolactin causes the mammary glands to synthesize and secrete milk, while oxytocin causes breast cells to contract, ejecting it. Oxytocin causes the uterus to contract as well. After a while, the mother might find that just thinking about the baby or hearing it cry triggers the oxytocin response, the "letdown reflex" (originally a dairy term—cows "let down" their udders for milking), with no stimulation of her nipples. By many accounts, oxytocin release and letdown are accompanied by a pleasant feeling of well-being and closeness to the child.

Two other reproduction-related events also trigger oxytocin release: childbirth and orgasm. Women release oxytocin when they give birth because it causes uterine contractions. Its role in orgasm probably derives not from its motor effects, however, but from its subjectively-perceived neurochemical effects. The feelings of closeness and well-being it elicits aid in pair-bonding. The more outward effects do assert themselves, however, and some nursing women, when they reach orgasm, release or even squirt jets of milk.

Breast-feeding also delays the return of ovulation and menses, helping to space children out at semi-manageable intervals. Nonlactating women typically ovulate four to six weeks after delivery, while women who nurse usually don't ovulate before four months have passed.

Semen

Semen. The one word, said in the right way, conjures up vivid images of strapping young sailors gaily frolicking above (or below) the deck of a ship. But wherever semen may appear, at sea, on land, or even in the air, it displays many unique characteristics. Semen is a fascinating, "living" liquid, and it's widely available.

The human male orgasm produces about 3.5 ml. of ejaculate, containing about 300 million spermatazoa zooming around in a complex liquid environment that protects and nourishes the hardiest among them for up to a couple of days. Aspiring nanotech engineers can learn a lot from the sperm's elegant design. A chemical process at the

base of its spiral-shaped tail causes the tail to rotate around like a propeller, powering the cell forward while converting fructose (fruit sugar) fuel from the surrounding liquid into lactic acid. As the tiny sperm courier their payloads of information, they alter the semen by rapidly depleting its sugar fuel level. Within one hour after ejaculation, 30% of the originally-motile sperm can no longer move. Within seven hours, half of them have stopped.

The general physical properties of semen also change. Upon delivery, semen is a thick liquid. It immediately begins to coagulate, however, and within five minutes it becomes a gel-like mass that, one expert notes, can be moved around as a single unit. Then it begins to re-liquefy, completely returning to the state of a free-flowing liquid in another twenty minutes. This coagulation and liquefaction takes place both *in vivo* and *in vitro*, but the semen liquefies faster in a vagina than in a room-temperature petri dish.

The coagulate phase temporarily immobilizes the sperm, and is thought to serve as a resting period that girds them for the second part of their journey. Where their path leads depends on external factors, but it begins in the testes, when oxytocin, the chemical which triggers milk ejection and cervical contraction in women, causes the semeniferous tubules to contract, launching the novice spermatozoa. The route continues past the prostate gland, the seminal vesicles, and Cowper's and Littré's glands, each of which makes its own contribution to the custom-mixed concoction, before leading out through the urethra and into the world.

The semen exits not as a uniform mix but as a series of liquids. The secretions from Cowper's and Littré's glands, which make up about 5% of the total volume, pave the way by lubricating the urethra during high arousal and early ejaculation. The prostatic fluid with the sperm mixed in, constituting about 25% of the volume, comes next, and finally, the largest component, the fluid from the misleadingly-named seminal vesicles (misleadingly named because they do not store semen, but, like the other glands, manufacture one of its components), brings up the rear. The vesicular secretion contains the sperms' bed and board, the coagulating agents and the fructose, along with most of the potassium and protein. Meanwhile, the liquefying enzymes, along with most of the cholesterol, citric acid, inositol, zinc, and magnesium, come from the prostatic fluid.

The resulting parfait is translucent whitish-grey in color, with a yellowish cast when produced after a long period of abstinence. Its odor resembles that of chestnut or carob flowers. Its chemistry varies widely, but in very rough numbers, 3.5 ml of semen contains 11 mg. carbohydrates, 150 mg. protein, 3% of the U.S. RDA for copper and zinc, 7% of the RDA for potassium, less than one calorie, and only 3 mg. cholesterol and 6 mg. fat.

Vaginal Secretions

Vaginal secretions contain many things, including sweat, sebum, and secretions from Bartholin's and Skene's glands at the vulva, endometrial and oviductal fluids (which change with the menstrual cycle), cervical mucus, exfoliated cells, and secretions of the vaginal walls themselves, which increase with sexual arousal. All women's vaginal secretions include pyridine, squalene, urea, acetic acid, lactic acid, complex alcohols (including cholesterol), glycols (including propylene glycol), ketones, and aldehydes.

But a more detailed chemistry of the acids in vaginal secretions separates women into two groups. All women produce acetic acid, but one third of them produce other short-chain aliphatic acids as well. The short-chain aliphatic acids, which include acetic, propionic, isovaleric, isobutyric, propanoic, and butanoic acids, are a pungent class of chemicals which other primate species produce as sexual-olfactory signals. Although no one has yet proven the acids' role in the mating behavior of humans, some researchers have referred to them "copulins" and "human pheromones."

Like the volatile acids produced on the skin, the vagina's aliphatic acids come from the metabolic processes of resident bacteria, including Lactobacilli, Streptococci, and Staphylococci. For

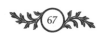

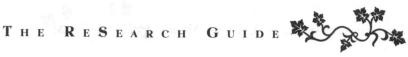

all women, the acid content varies with the menstrual cycle, rising from day one after menstruation and peaking at mid-cycle, just before ovulation. The amounts vary more dramatically in the acid producers, however, and one study, whose authors describe their subjects as "young, healthy, and members of the socioeconomic class that attends a privately endowed university," determined that people can reliably smell changes in an acid-producing woman's vaginal secretions over the course of her cycle, but not in the secretions of a non-acid producer.

Female Ejaculate

Many women report that they release a liquid from their urethras when they have an orgasm, usually describing it as a small spurt of something thinner than regular vaginal secretions. Some of the women assume that it's simply urine, while others believe it to be something else, a distinct female ejaculate. During the past decade, however, a good number of researchers have studied the issue, and as a result of their findings, some of them believe that it's simply urine, while others believe it to be a distinct female ejaculate.

Urinary incontinence at orgasm in some women has been well-documented, and chemical tests of female ejaculate, pure samples of which are difficult to collect, show it to be similar to urine, but possibly containing extra ingredients from Skene's glands, small glands considered to be female homologues to the prostate, which empty into the urethra near its exit. Given our current knowledge (or lack thereof), you can make cases for calling the liquid that some women release at orgasm from their urethras either "female ejaculate" or "urine," depending on what you want to call it, or which set of associations or images you prefer.

Sebum

Sebum, or skin oil, functions to reduce moisture loss through our skin, protect it from infections, and lubricate it in contact areas. It also makes hair shiny and waterproof and helps generate scents. Sebaceous glands occur all over the skin, except for the palms and soles, and are largest and most numerous on the back, forehead, face, ears, genitals, and anal region. Most connect to hair follicles, but some, such as the Meibomian glands (in the eyelids), Tyson's glands (in the foreskin), and the sebaceous glands around the nipples and along the edge of the upper lip, empty directly onto the surface of the skin. On some people, you can see the ones along the lip as pale yellow specks, or "Fordyce's spots."

Sebum consists of 57.5% glycerides and free fatty acids, 26% wax esters, 12% squalene, 3% cholesterol esters, and 1.5% cholesterol, but despite its fatty, waxy content, sebum production does not correlate with dietary fat intake. However, it does correlate with levels of testosterone and other androgens. Men produce more sebum than women and prepubertal boys, and uncastrated men produce more than eunuchs. Male sebum production increases fivefold during puberty, causing acne. But interestingly, newborns secrete sebum at adult levels for a short time after birth, and women secrete greater amounts during pregnancy and lactation.

Menses

As you may recall from Sex Ed in Junior High, humans differ from most other mammals in that they're fully equipped to mate and reproduce all year long, and not just during an annual or semi-annual mating season. To help accomplish this, the pituitary gland times the cyclic release of estrogen, progesterone, and follicle stimulating hormone (FSH). During ovulation, triggered by FSH, an ovary pushes an egg into its fallopian tube. If the egg is fertilized, it imbeds in the uterine lining, the endometrium, and pregnancy commences. Otherwise, the climbing progesterone level eventually signals the uterus to contract and discard its contents, enabling the system to begin again.

Blood comprises about two thirds of these contents. The rest consists mainly of mucus and frag-

ments of the uterine mucous membrane, which picks up some scaling cell tissues from the vagina on the way out. The resulting menstrual fluid also differs from circulating blood in that it contains much more lime and lacks the ability to clot. One recent article points out that the uterine lining can also contain pathogens introduced by sperm, and that menstruation works to clear the pathogens out.

Anorexia, heroin addiction, tuberculosis, radiation sickness, and other diseases can halt the cycle, as will pregnancy and menopause, but otherwise it continues through much of a woman's life, and in the absence of artificial lighting can even synchronize with phases of the moon: ovulation at full moon and menstruation at new moon is considered the natural rhythm. Synchronization also occurs among women living together, a phenomenon known as the McClintock effect, due to chemicals contained in sweat. When the sweat of one woman is regularly deposited beneath the nose of a second woman she has no other contact with, the second woman's cycle will synchronize with the first's within three months.

During ovulation, women see and hear better, are less bothered by physical pain, and are more likely to be elated. Two weeks earlier or later, at menstruation, they're more prone to skin conditions such as herpes, acne, and dark circles under the eyes and more susceptible to vaginal infections. Some menstruating women also develop "menses breath," an oniony smell from balance changes in the body's sulfur compounds, and some report a special desire to tidy up.

Some evidence shows that men also have a menstrual cycle affecting mood and alertness, and one Japanese railway company significantly increased productivity and reduced accidents after trying to fit their (male) drivers' work schedules to match these cycles. But swings in temperament are far less obvious than menstrual bleeding, so any mysterious monthly cycling has generally been associated solely with women. The ways people in a culture regard and deal with this "female" trait often reflect the culture's dominant attitudes towards women as a whole.

Early societies must have pondered the menstrual cycle and felt awe at how it seemed connected to the moon, how it deferred only to old age and wisdom or to the greater mystery of pregnancy and birth, how it reflected the seasons and the eternal cycles of fertility and growth, birth and death, how it yielded blood, life's essence, which otherwise came only with disease or injury and yet left the woman unharmed. Many ancient religions revered women as fertile creators connected to the rhythms of the universe and its (usually female) Creator, and communities relied on the wisdom and guidance of post-menopausal women leaders.

These older, more matriarchal societies worshipped primeval mother creator gods such as Tiamat of the Mesopotamians and Lilith of the Sumerians. Stone Age cave paintings in Africa and Europe depict menstruation, and the earliest calendars, prehistoric notched bones and pegboards, are traditionally thought to be menstrual calendars used to worship Tiamat, who according to legend created the earth from her menstrual blood. Older cultures, and many modern indigenous cultures as well, surround menstruation and especially the menarche with ritual and worship. The young woman coming of age will often leave the community for days or even years before returning as a newly eligible, fertile young adult. Possibly originally in imitation of menarche, young men's initiation rituals often include circumcision, subincision, or other bloody forms of genital mutilation. Wogeo Islander men of New Guinea incise their penises periodically, simulating not just menarche but regular menstruation.

In parts of Eastern Europe, families announce a daughter's first menses more informally, by hanging the stained bedsheets out the window, in the same manner as some Mediterranean families seek to confirm their daughters' maidenhood at marriage the morning after. Some cultures directly equate hymenal and menstrual blood by explaining menarche as evidence of the young woman's defloration by an aerial spirit.

Another widespread set of traditions secludes the menstruating woman in a special area away from the community for the duration of her pe-

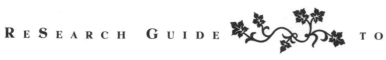

riod. Depending on the culture's view of women, this menstrual hut is seen as a sacred place for a time during which the woman communed with the ancestors and the universe before returning with new perspectives and plans, or else as an exile during which the menstruating woman, with her poisonous blood, poisonous breath, and evil eye, could be kept safely out of the way to avoid bringing bad luck to the vulnerable village.

In *Dragontime* (1991), German author and screenwriter Luisa Francia recommends that women revive some of the old menstrual rituals and set up menstrual "huts" or altars in their own homes. For her and for many women she knows, doing this has eased the pain and nuisance of menstruation and turned it into a special "away" time, a monthly vacation from modern life allowing them to reconnect with tradition, nature, and themselves. She envisions menstrual huts set up in cities today, cozy havens where menstruating women could go to relax, talk, read, write, drink herb tea and hot cocoa, and eat hot soup. (I myself can imagine such places succeeding wonderfully in all major U.S. cities, as well as smaller ones like Berkeley, Northampton, Ann Arbor, Boulder, Austin, and Madison.)

Francia also recommends visiting old sacred menstrual sites during menstruation. You can find them, she says, at springs near caves or small chapels, and their folk names often include "Mary's," "Women's," "Hell's," or "Witches." Of these sites, she writes, "with fear of making good anthropologists howl. . .I must confess that it's very exciting to engage in little rituals in places already enlivened by folklore."

Women of various cultures have also dealt with the menstrual blood itself in various ways. Before the twentieth century brought modern napkins, tampons, and pads, women in the U.S. and Europe used thick cotton cloth diaper/napkin/bandage type undergarments which they washed and reused. In Africa and Australia, the cloth bandages were made of grass or vegetable fiber. Japanese women used paper tampons and held them in place with bandages. Indonesians made tampons from vegetable fiber. The Romans used

soft wool. The Egyptians used rolls of soft papyrus. Equatorial Africans used rolls of grass and roots. Meanwhile, the Tuareg women of the Sahara didn't use anything at all, and still don't. When their periods begin, they dig a hole in the ground and squat over it to let the first flow out. After this, they tense their muscles to hold it in and can regulate the bleeding in this way throughout the menstruation. If a small trickle escapes inadvertently, they simply spread their legs wide and it quickly dries out in the desert air. They wear no underpants and jump and move around from time to time to help air out their vaginas. As a result, Luisa Francia notes, they never get the light odor of stale blood common among Europeans.

Almost as common as menstruation itself are menstrual taboos. The word "taboo" itself, in fact, probably evolved from "tupua," a Polynesian word for menstruation. The traditional menstrual taboos as we know them purport to protect the men and the crops rather than the women themselves, and forbid far more than sex. Many cultures fear and isolate menstruating women, or prevent them from planting, harvesting, and cooking. Any contact with menstrual blood itself is likewise feared, and our own superstition that walking under ladders brings bad luck comes from the idea that a menstruating woman might be on the ladder.

Judeo-Christian-Islamic writings and tradition strongly tabooed menstruation, and just as they demonized scatological practices of pagan origin, they associated menstruation and menstrual rites with witchcraft and evil (that witchcraft and evil are associated in the first place is itself a patriarchal editorialization.). The Bible defines menstruating women and their blood as unclean (Leviticus 15:19-33) and characterizes them as loathsome (Genesis 31:35, Isaiah 30:22, Esther 14:16), and while intellectual Christian men during the Middle Ages debated whether or not menstruating women should be allowed to enter churches and receive communion, their more action-oriented brothers were busy trying, torturing, and killing as witches any women who held

onto remnants of the more evenly-empowering older religions institutional Christianity had an interest in stamping out.

This displacement of older, nature-worshipping, polytheistic religions by newer, monotheistic, patriarchal ones like Christianity reveals itself through myths and folklore. In the Babylonian myth of earth-mother Tiamat, one of Tiamat's sons, Marduk, attacks Tiamat to take her power away. In the earliest versions of the myth Tiamat eats Marduk, but in later versions, Marduk splits Tiamat in half with his sword, kills her and successfully gains her power. In Greek mythology, Zeus gives birth to Athena out of his head, illustrating how men deal with womb envy by creating things with their brains, creating "brain children." Christian hagiography has several accounts of male saints battling and slaying dragons, which Francia suggests symbolize menstruating women and paganism/witchcraft. Menstruating women and dragons, Francia argues, both have an evil eye, a deadly touch, and hot, poisonous breath, and both seek almandites, or bloodstones, known as dragonstones in myth, precious red stones traditionally thought to help with menstrual problems. Folk tales such as Cinderella, Rose Red, and Rapunzel contain symbols of menstruation and menarcheal seclusion: bloodied feet, thorn-pricked fingers, and isolated towers.

Psychologists, anthropologists, and others have proposed several explanations for the menstruation taboo. Freud ascribes it to a general fear of blood. Bettelheim suggests that men use it to compensate for their womb envy and to equalize the sexes. Others suggest that it comes from fear and reverence for the powers of nature. Certain, however, is that the taboo has persisted into recent times and the present despite invalidating scientific evidence. In the 19th century, Saigon's opium industry hired only men out of a fear that the proximity of a menstruating woman would make the product bitter and weak. An urban legend popular during the 1920's held that a perm would not "take" if the woman was menstruating at the time. Some German computer centers and pharmaceutical labs today require menstruating women to wear a red dot on their lab coats and bar their access to certain areas. During the twenties, a few scientists felt compelled to find a biological basis for the menstrual taboo. Bela Schick, developer of the Schick test for diphtheria immunity, sought to prove the existence of hypothesized "menotoxins," chemicals he thought exuded from the skin of menstruating women and harmed plant life, causing, for example, the wilting of flowers. Schick's hypotheses were soon discredited.

Anthropology has also been used as a platform to reinforce cultural prejudices regarding menstruation. Old-school armchair anthropologists once viewed menarcheal age as an indicator of "refinement" or "advancement." They argued that more hot-blooded, dark, primitive, and sexually precocious peoples typically had earlier average menarches. We now know that early menarche correlates with good nutrition, explaining why in this country each generation since 1850 has matured about one year earlier than the last. The "savages" the anthropologists wrote about were no more hot-blooded than were their daughters back home, but they may have had a healthier diet.

The twenties was an important decade for menstruation in a positive sense as well, however. During World War I, French nurses had discovered that bandage cellulose, made from wood pulp, absorbed menstrual blood better than cotton cloth. The product that resulted, Kotex sanitary napkins, hit the U.S. market in 1921, and all but replaced cloth "diapers" within a generation. Meanwhile, a leader of the Women's movement in the twenties, Clelia Duel Mosher, made the then-revolutionary argument in her *Health and the Woman Movement* and *Women's Physical Freedom*, that it is only through custom, the wishes of men, and the power of suggestion that people consider menstruation incapacitating, the "woman's lot" that has to be endured while resting at home, and that by simply changing their attitudes and, if necessary, abandoning cramp-aggravating fashions such as heavy skirts and tight corsets, women can feel and be every bit as capable of full-time work as men.

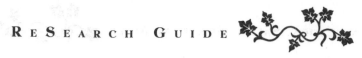
The next big innovation came with the Tampax tampon, made from expandable rayon, introduced in 1933. Despite the lingering issue of the carelessly-inserted tampon's ability to, in a crude sense, spoil a woman's virginity, the product became and continues to be a success.

Advertisements for feminine protection products first appeared in women's magazines in the thirties. They became more matter-of-fact and practical in tone during the forties, when most women worked for the war effort, but the fifties saw the return of coy language and condescension. Radio and television first carried tampon and pad ads in 1972.

Companies are still looking for a better way to contain menstrual flow, knowing that the profit potential is enormous. In 1969 a California company introduced the Tassaway, a flexible, nonabsorbent cup which fit into the vagina, but it didn't catch on. Work has also been done on suction tube "period extraction," a.k.a. "the fifteen minute period," but as yet it's risky and unproven, and people are understandably leery of making such an unnatural procedure a monthly routine.

Meanwhile, the environmental cost of disposable tampons and pads has prompted many women to experiment with less wasteful, homemade solutions. One author has had success with cutting a 3.5" by 4.5" synthetic sponge widthwise into four equal strips and using these as tampons, sterilizing them for reuse by boiling. Some health food stores now sell a reusable cloth sanitary napkin.

Sweat

Inspiration and perspiration—the two constituents of genius, according to Edison—also distinguish our species. Humans surpass nearly all other animals in the areas of brain power and ability to sweat, and we have pitted these two titans against one another in a battle so ferocious that its weapons—aerosol deodorants and air conditioning systems (which contain the chemical Freon)—have threatened the planet's ozone layer.

Only mammals sweat, and for all mammals except humans, horses, some cows, and the Patas monkey, sweating is just a way to lubricate footpads and other contact surfaces or to give off a scent. For the few exceptions, ourselves included, sweating also works as a cooling mechanism, and to this feature as much as to our intelligence we owe our adaptability to a variety of terrains and climates.

Life on earth originated in the ocean, and as Diane Ackerman points out (in *The Natural History of the Senses*, 1990), we land animals still carry the salty sea around within ourselves. Salt remains the main osmotic ingredient of our blood and extracellular fluid, and if we lose too much of it, we risk circulatory collapse. Most mammals are not equipped to sweat without freely losing salt, but our sweat glands conserve salt, and this is what enables us to run marathons, haul blocks of stone up uncompleted pyramids, and kill each other in tank battles in the hot desert sun.

The adult body contains from two to four million sweat glands, at densities of around one to two hundred per square centimeter of skin. Together, they typically put out from one to three quarts of perspiration per day, although a day of exertion and thirst-quenching in the heat can make a body sweat out fifteen quarts or more.

Most of our sweat glands are eccrine glands, the salt-retaining cooling sweat glands, most prevalent on the back, chest, forehead, palms, and soles. But we have another, older type of sweat gland, apocrine, which helps produce scents used for personal identification and mating. These scent glands concentrate most highly in the underarms, but also surround the nipples, genitals, and anus, and as many have noticed, they respond to stress. Apocrine sweat contains an odor resembling musk, a substance secreted as a scent by deer and other animals and used in perfume. This has led some observers to remark that our toilet ritual has us wash away our own sweat and substitute the sweat of deer. An experiment conducted at International Flavors and Fragrances in New York showed that women who sniff musk develop shorter menstrual cycles, ovulate more

often, and conceive more easily.

Apocrine sweat has no odor when it arrives on the skin surface, but it is immediately broken down by bacteria, including Staphylococcus epidermis (the most prevalent), S. saprophyticus (more prevalent in winter), S. aureus (more prevalent in summer), Escherichia coli, and various species of Corynebacteria, Brevibacteria, Propionibacteria (more prevalent in men), Enterobacter, Klebsiella, and Proteus. These flora generate compounds such as androstenone ("stale urine" smell), androstenol (nice "musky" odor), and isovaleric acid (sweaty or "goatlike" smell).

The prehistoric invention of clothing had the sometime effect of limiting air circulation to underarms and the rest of the body, intensifying apocrine "body odor." Extreme body odor has been considered disagreeable for centuries (Ovid mentions it), but people experience normal amounts (relative to cultural norms) as reassuring and even sexy. In a letter, Napoleon once asked Josephine not to bathe during the two weeks that would pass before they met again.

Our culture tolerates sweat odors much less than it used to, however. Specific products for the underarm first appeared only about a century ago, and today, over 90% of the U.S. adult population uses a deodorant or antiperspirant daily. The past century has seen a parade of product innovations devoted to this few square inches of skin.

The first trademarked brand was 1888's Mum, a waxy zinc oxide deodorant cream. The first true antiperspirant, Everdry, a solution of aluminum chloride in water, appeared around 1900. Early aluminum chloride products—liquids dabbed on with cotton—felt sticky and cold and often irritated or stung. The only group to fully embrace the products were entertainers, but in 1914, Odo-Ro-No did become popular enough to support national advertising.

The 30's brought antiperspirants based on aluminum sulfate: sticks based on soap and emollient oils and creams such as 1934's Arrid Cream. The sticks felt greasy and never caught on widely, but the creams were as easy to apply as the already existing deodorant creams, and they be-

came the dominant type of product until the mid-40's, which brought liquid-soaked pads in jars (5-Day Deodorant Pads) and squeezable plastic spray bottles (Stoppette Spray Deodorant). The plastic spray bottle allowed users to apply the product without getting it on their fingers, but the product took a while to dry and often dripped.

In 1947, non-stinging aluminum chlorohydrate began to replace the aluminum salts in antiperspirants. In 1952, Mum Roullette came out, the first roll-on (inspired by the ball-point pen). It didn't work quite as well as the later Ban Roll-On (1955), and so it faded away.

In the early 60's, Gillette introduced Right Guard deodorant, the first aerosol. The finer spray and quicker drying time compared to squeeze bottles made it an immediate success. Five years later, after problems with clogging had been overcome, the first aerosol anti-perspirant came out, but in the mid to late 70's, the FDA started questioning the safety of aluminum and zirconium salts in aerosols, particularly when inhaled daily for years, and the public began realizing that the aerosol propellants were destroying the ozone layer.

The industry switched to hydrocarbon propellants and the FDA banned zirconium-based antiperspirants. Meanwhile, the sensible public largely switched away from aerosols to less wasteful delivery methods. A new type of pump spray came out in the 70's, and the development of volatile silicones, which evaporate without feeling cool, enabled the introduction of an improved antiperspirant roll-on (Dry Idea, 1978) and improved deodorant and antiperspirant sticks (such as Mennen Deodorant Stick) that are less greasy than their 30's forebears. These types have become the most popular. Health food stores now carry "natural" deodorant crystals to combat armpit odor while contributing no scent of their own.

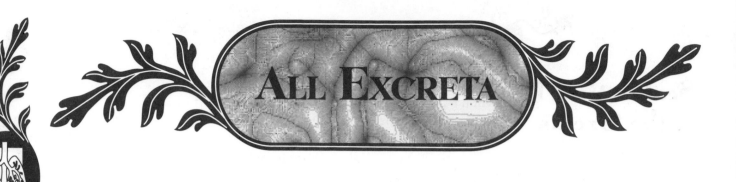

ALL EXCRETA

Excreta
DEJECTA, EGESTA, EXCREMENT, EXCRETIONS

Toilet/Toilet Room
CRAPPER, CAN, JOHN, JAKES, BIFFY, DOOLEY, DUNNY, DUFFS, CARSEY, DONNICKER, FLUSHER, AJAX, CLOSE STOOL, COMMODE, HEAD, LATRINE, LAVATORY, LAVABO, LAV, LOO, PAN, POT, POTTY, THRONE, CONVENIENCE, FACILITY, CHIC SALE, DOINGS, PRIVY, BOG, NECESSARIUM, GARDEROBE, GEOGRAPHY, HOLY OF HOLIES

Rooms, Houses, Etc.
MEN'S/WOMEN'S/LADIES'/LITTLE BOYS' ROOM, REST ROOM, BATHROOM, OUTHOUSE, WATER CLOSET, WC, EARTH CLOSET, COMMON HOUSE, COMFORT STATION, CLOAK ROOM, SHOT TOWER, SMALLEST ROOM, PENNY-HOUSE, CHAMBER OF COMMERCE, THE HOUSE OF HONOR, THE HOUSE OF THE MORNING, NECESSARY HOUSE, PLACE OF EASEMENT, THE PROVERBIAL BRICK SHITHOUSE/OUTHOUSE, NUMERO CENTO (ITALY)

Go To The Toilet (any phrase will work, but these are more common:)
BE EXCUSED, PICK A DAISY, SEE THE GEOGRAPHY OF THE HOUSE, WASH YOUR HANDS, TURN YOUR BICYCLE AROUND, SEE A MAN ABOUT A DOG, GO TO THE DIKE, GO TELEPHONE HITLER (POPULAR AMONG WWII FRENCH RESISTANCE)

In many areas of knowledge, as in sewers, it's not worth the trouble to separate different types of excreta away from one another. They're all mixed in together as a whole. At a general level, we view our body products as all the same (reminders of our animal natures, of mortality, of poverty, of our unity with the earth, etc.), and so the technologies, social constructs, and artistic/literary themes they have sparked are similar or identical. Polite society hides and ignores boogers just as it hides and ignores sweat and shit. Our great invention the toilet (along with the sewer infrastructure it connects to) whisks away urine, feces, vomit, menstrual blood, and mucus alike, and it stands right near similar fixtures which take care of sweat, saliva, and other excreta.

The general category of All Excreta has a wider influence than any one excretion alone, covering history, technology, psychology, religion, medicine, custom, literature, the arts, industry, design, architecture, folklore, and even gastronomy.

Scatological Lives of the Greats

In *Works and Days*, 8th century B.C. Greek poet **Hesiod** recommended peeing seated or against a wall rather than out in the open.

Aesop (620?-560?), upon seeing his master urinate while walking, and lamenting the quickening pace of life in Ancient Greece: "What next? Will we have to shit as we run?"

Cynic philosopher **Diogenes** (412?-323) thought modesty was absurd and that what could be done privately without shame could just as well be done without shame in public. To prove his point, it is said, he routinely defecated in the marketplace.

Stoic philosopher **Crates** (flourished 328-324) rid Peripatetic philosopher **Metrocles** of his concern for politeness, drawing him over to Stoicism, by initiating a farting contest with him.

According to legend, the sweat of **Alexander the Great** (356-323) had a sweet odor.

In *The Art of Love*, **Ovid** (Publius Ovidius Naso 43 B.C.-A.D. 17?) advises people looking for love to control their body odor, telling them, "I warn you that no rude goat find its way beneath your arms."

The first thing **Johannes Gutenberg** (1400?-1468) printed after his Bible was the "Laxierkalender" (1457), a calendar that indicated the best times and dates to use laxatives.

Joan of Arc (1412?-1431), who died young but not *that* young, is said to have never menstruated.

In *Utopia* by **Sir Thomas More** (1478-1535), chamber-pots were made of gold and silver, preventing citizens from revering the metals. In 1523, More wrote to **Martin Luther** that as long as Luther kept spouting lies, England would permit others "to throw back into your. . .shitty mouth, truly the shit-pool of all shit, all the muck and shit which your damnable rottenness has vomited up, and to empty out all the sewers and privies onto your crown."

Martin Luther (1483-1546) suffered constipation and tended to speak, write, and think in scatological imagery. He got his initial Protestant inspiration, the "revelation in the tower" that salvation comes through faith alone and has nothing to do with the organized church, while defecating. He described visions of an anus-faced **Satan** mooning him and farting on him and described the Pope and the Catholic Church in similarly scatological terms.

Richard III (1452-1485), king of England and subject of **William Shakespeare's** play, plotted his nephews' murders with **Terril** while seated on the close-stool.

Charles V (1500-1558), king of Spain and emperor of the Holy Roman Empire was born in a latrine.

In "Of vanity," **Michel Eyquem Montaigne** (1533-1592) describes his *Essays* as "some excrements of an aged mind, now hard, now loose, and always undigested." Here are some choice leavings:

(Of the power of the imagination:) "The organs that serve to discharge the stomach have their own dilations and compressions, beyond and against our plans, just like those that are destined to discharge the kidneys . . . . I know one so turbulent and unruly, that for forty years it has kept its master farting with a constant and unremitting wind and compulsion, and is thus taking him to his death."

(Of vanity:) "I knew a gentleman who gave knowledge of his life only by the workings of his belly; you should see on display at his home a row of chamber pots, seven or eight days' worth. That was his study, his conversation; all other talk stank in his nostrils."

(Of experience:) "Both kings and philosophers defecate, and ladies too . . . . Wherefore I will say this about that action: that we should relegate it to certain prescribed nocturnal hours, and force and subject ourselves to them by habit . . . . Of all natural functions that is the one that I can least willingly endure to have interrupted. I have seen many soldiers inconvenienced by the irregularity of their bowels; mine and I never fail the moment of our assignation, which is when I

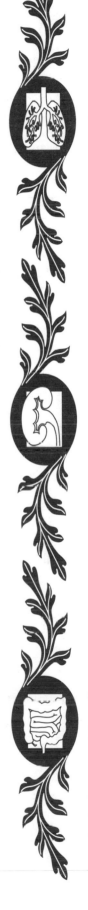

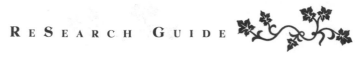

jump out of bed."

(Of experience:) "I do not remember ever having had the itch; yet scratching is one of the sweetest gratifications of nature, and as ready at hand as any. But repentance follows too annoyingly close at its heels. I mostly scratch my ears, which are sometimes itchy on the inside."

Popular legend has it that **Sir Walter Raleigh** (1552?-1618) placed his coat over a puddle of urine in **Queen Elizabeth I**'s path to obviate her need to walk around it.

Sir Francis Bacon (1561-1626): "Money is like manure, very little use except it be spread."

James I (1566-1625), king of England, Ireland, and Scotland, reportedly enjoyed hunting so much that he routinely shat in his pants rather than interrupt the hunt.

Pioneer physicist/chemist **Robert Boyle** (1627-1691) recommended enemas of tobacco smoke and eye lotions of powdered human feces ("**Paracelsus**'s Zibethum Occidentale").

Louis XIV (1638-1715), king of France, loved enemas.

Belletrist **Liselotte** (Elizabeth Charlotte of the Palatinate, 1652-1722), of the court of **Louis XIV**, in a letter to her aunt in Hanover (1694): "You are fortunate to be able to shit when you wish. Shit then to your heart's content. We are not in the same situation here where I am obliged to keep my shitload until evening . . . . It is extremely depressing that my pleasures are impeded by piles of shit. I wish that he who invented shitting, I wish that he and all his kin would be able to shit only by having it beaten out of them . . . . I know of nothing more disgusting than shitting. You see a beautiful person, neat, clean, you cry out, 'how charming it would be if she didn't shit!' . . . . If you think you are kissing a pretty little mouth with all white teeth—you are kissing a shitmill: Every single delicacy, biscuits, pastries, tarts, fillings, hams, partridges, pheasants, etc. all of it exists only to be made into ground up shit."

Jonathan Swift (1667-1745) suggested that philosophers and statesmen should care for privies, to better have a handle on the condition of the country. His many scatologically oriented writings are literary landmarks.

François Voltaire (1694-1778), panicked on his death bed, reached into the chamberpot and ate.

After the Royal Academy of Brussels belittled some of **Benjamin Franklin**'s (1706-1790) discoveries, he wrote them a letter suggesting that they begin researching how to render the scent of farts pleasant to others, arguing that succeeding would improve people's lives more than any of the discoveries of Aristotle, Descartes, and Newton ("What comfort can the vortices of Descartes give to a man who has whirlwinds in his bowels!"). He never sent the letter.

Lexicographer **Samuel Johnson** (1709-1784): "Much has been written of the pleasures of sexual intercourse, as for me, give me a solid movement of the bowel."

Wolfgang Amadeus Mozart (1756-1791) composed vocal canons around the texts "Lick my ass" ("Leck mich im Arsch," the closest German equivalent to our "Fuck you"), and "Lick my ass nice and clean." He also included phrases such as "I shit in your mouth" in some of his longer works. He wrote about scatological subjects in his letters as well, one of which he signed, with characteristic egotism, "W. A. Mozart, who shits without a fart."

British general **Sir John Moore** (1761-1809), according to Captain **John Gregory Bourke**, "fell in love with his own urine." Bourke gives no further details.

George Gordon, Lord Byron (1788-1824) suggested as the epitaph for **Robert Steward, Viscount Castlereagh**:

"Posterity will ne'er survey
A nobler grave than this
Here lie the bones of Castlereagh
Stop, traveler, ____"

Honoré de Balzac (1799-1850): "I should like one of these days to be so well-known, so popular, so celebrated, so famous, that it would permit me to break wind in society and society would think it a most natural thing."

James Joyce (1822-1941), in a letter to his wife, **Nora**: "The smallest things give me a great

cockstand. . .a little brown stain on the seat of your white drawers. . .a sudden immodest noise made by you behind and then a bad smell slowly curling up out of your backside. I hope Nora will let off no end of farts in my face so that I may know their smell also. It must be a fearfully lecherous thing to see a girl with her clothes up frigging furiously at her cunt, to see her pretty white drawers pulled open behind and her bum sticking out and a fat brown thing stuck halfway out of her hole."

As a youth, **Thomas Alva Edison** (1847-1931) fed his playmate **Michael Oates** large doses of a laxative to see if Michael could then fly through the air under the power of his farts.

Sigmund Freud (1856-1939) frequently suffered from constipation.

George Bernard Shaw (1856-1950) on **Chic Sale**'s scatological humor bestseller *The Specialist:* "The illustrations are excellent; but the frontispiece fails in courage. Clearly it should represent the Elmer family *in situ*. G. B. S."

As a young man, **William Randolph Hearst** (1863-1951) sent to several teachers he disliked chamberpots with their pictures pasted in the bottoms. He was expelled from school.

Mahatma Mohandas Gandhi (1869-1948) used to ask his female attendants, "Did you have a good bowel movement this morning, sister?"

In 1906, **Maxfield Parrish** (1870-1966) painted a mural for the bar room of the Knickerbocker Hotel in New York that depicted Old King Cole, legend has it, in the act of farting.

John Cowper Powys (1872-1963) read through all of **Rabelais** and two volumes of **Montaigne** while on the toilet.

The house of **Winston Churchill** (1874-1965) at Hyde Park Gate had seats on the guests' toilets, but none on his own. When the plumber suggested he could fit a seat onto Churchill's toilet, he replied, "I have no need of such things."

In *On a Chinese Screen*, **W. Somerset Maugham** (1874-1965) describes how equality of hygiene in China results in the upper and lower classes there interacting more closely than they do in the West. He goes on to write, as Orwell quotes, "In the West

we are divided from our fellows by our sense of smell . . . . The matutinal tub divides the classes more effectually than birth, wealth or education."

In his memoirs, pioneer psychologist **Carl Jung** (1875-1961) writes that at age twelve, he became obsessed with the image of **God** sitting on a golden throne in the sky above a cathedral. The image frightened him until he finally imagined an enormous turd fall down from underneath the throne and break through the roof of the cathedral. At that moment, he realized that **God** did not want him to limit his thinking.

According to *Newsweek* (9 July 1973), **Joseph Stalin** (1879-1953) tried to cover up the sound of his farts "by rattling the water carafe and glasses he kept on his desk."

Adolf Hitler (1889-1945), troubled by chronic, uncontrollable farting, took charcoal pills and even nonlethal amounts of strychnine and belladonna in attempts to control the gas.

In a back room during the Nuremberg Trials, **Hermann Wilhelm Göring** (1893-1946) pounded his fist on a table and explained that he wished he and his associates had the strength and moral conviction to answer every single question asked of them on the witness stand with "Leck mich im Arsch" ("Lick my ass").

Mao Zedong (1893-1976) frequently suffered constipation, and routinely had his bodyguards pry feces from his anus with their fingers. Constipation made Mao irritable and affected his decisions, and when a long bout of constipation ended for him, word would spread through the relieved government, "The chairman's bowels have moved! He had a good shit!" For years, Mao preferred going into fields to defecate over using an indoor toilet, explaining that the toilet's odor got in the way of his thinking. He viewed dung as a symbol of purity and peasant virtue, and branded those who didn't want to handle it as intellectuals and parasites.

According to legend, **George Herman "Babe" Ruth** (1895-1948) refused a plate of asparagus at a fancy dinner with the line, "No thanks, ma'am. That stuff makes my farts smell awful!"

Yves Tanguy (1900-1955) was, at least accord-

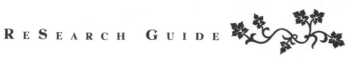

ing to rival Surrealist **Salvador Dali**, "the greatest petomaniac of his time. He was capable of putting out a candle at a distance of two yards simply by bending over in a certain way. He even played pool with his farts." Of himself, Dali writes, "I cannot help noticing that I hardly fart at all."

In his handbook on how to live an Islamically Correct life in the modern world, *Worship and Self-Development According to the Tahrir al-Wasilah of Ayatollah 'Uzma Imam Khomeini*, **The Ayatollah Ruhollah Khomeini** (1900-1989) writes: "Where there are Western toilets (which do not have the necessary equipment to purify oneself), one can use either the French bidet, if there is one, or a hose or a container with a spout like a watering can or a kettle and purify oneself with water. Or (in the case of feces), one can purify oneself with toilet paper just as one can purify oneself with a stone or a clot of earth or a piece of cloth. In such a case, the criteria is the removal of the ritual impurity . . . . It is not necessary that one purify one's self with three cloths, for three sides of one stone or cloth are enough. Furthermore, if the ritual impurity is removed with one wiping, this is sufficient and the criteria is its removal, but the outlet of urine becomes purified only with water."

George Orwell (1903-1950), in *The Road to Wigan Pier* (1937): ". . .Here you come to the real secret of class distinctions in the West—the real reason why a European of bourgeois upbringing, even when he calls himself a Communist, cannot without a hard effort think of a working man as his equal. It is summed up in four frightful words which people nowadays are chary of uttering, but which were bandied about quite freely in my childhood. The words were: *The lower classes smell.*"

In his *Diary of a Genius* (1965), many entries in which discuss strange dreams about turds and morning turds themselves, **Salvador Dali** (1904-1982) writes: "Temporal immortality must be looked for in refuse, in excrement and nowhere else . . . . I am dumbfounded by how little philosophical and metaphysical importance the human mind has attached to the capital subject of excrement." In *The Secret Life of Salvador Dali* (1942), he relates that he once went into a panic because

he thought a piece of dried mucus under his fingernail was going to kill him ("All that I had needed, in order to descend into 'hell,' was a piece of mucus.").

Howard Hughes (1905-1976) suffered from constipation and once spent three continuous days on the toilet dozing, waking, and waiting.

Lyndon Baines Johnson (1908-1973) was, according to **David Halberstam**, "the earthiest man in the White House in a century." Halberstam writes that LBJ routinely demanded that associates accompany him to the bathroom to continue meetings while he defecated, a habit which particularly annoyed Treasury Secretary **Douglas Dillon.** Discussing a potential staffer, he demanded, "I don't want loyalty. I want *loyalty*. I want him to kiss my ass in Macy's window at high noon and tell me it smells like roses." On Congress, he complained, "They'll push Vietnam up my ass every time. Vietnam. Vietnam. Vietnam. Right up my ass." On a member of his administration who was turning into a dove: "Hell, he has to squat to piss." On a speech by **Richard Nixon**: "I may not know much but I know the difference between chicken shit and chicken salad." On getting rid of **J. Edgar Hoover**: "Well, it's probably better to have him inside the tent pissing out, than outside pissing in." Unrelatedly, Johnson would also freely reach over with his fork and eat off of other people's plates.

Katharine Hepburn (1909-), in *The Making of The African Queen*: "Bowels are not exactly a polite subject for conversation, but they are certainly a common problem . . . please think of me again as the urologist's daughter . . . . It may disgust you that I have brought it up at all, but who knows? Life has some problems which are basic for all of us—and about which we have a natural reticence."

British physicist **Reginald V. Jones** (1911-) won a barracks contest by peeing over a six foot wall.

Dylan Thomas (1914-1953) suggested that novels be serialized on rolls of toilet paper.

Television host **Jack Paar** (1918-) first met television-host-to-be **Dick Cavett** in a men's room, and hired him shortly thereafter. Paar told people that had he had his own private bathroom at NBC at the time, Dick Cavett wouldn't be around today.

During his 8 January 1992 dinner at the official residence of **Kiichi Miyazawa**, **George Bush** (1924-), suffering intestinal flu, vomited and collapsed. He left the residence in a green overcoat provided by a Secret Service agent to cover his stained clothes. The incident inspired a new Japanese slang term for vomiting: *bushusuru*.

Lenny Bruce (Leonard Schneider 1925-1966) writes that in 1951, at the beginning of his comedy career, established show-biz types frequently told him, "You'll go a long way, Lenny; you're funny and clean." Over the next decade, however, he steered toward more controversial material, and in October 1961 he was arrested for public obscenity, immediately following a San Francisco performance in which he used the word "cocksucker" and the phrases "Did you come good?" and "Don't come in me." The case went to trial and Bruce was found not guilty, but he soon faced a series of arrests in other cities, for both obscenity and drug possession, and he spent much of the rest of his life fighting the legal battles that resulted.

Idi Amin Dada (1925-) imprisoned a cameraman and a studio technician after a television newscast showed him greeting a foreign dignitary by offering his left hand.

Singer **Tiny Tim** (Herbert Khaury, 1927-) in *Esquire* (Dec. 1970): "I take one big shower a day and then a shower, soaping three times, every time nature calls. This is not to offend the public, it avoids stains on the underwear and it gives a feeling of security."

Madonna (Madonna Ciccone, 1958-): "Sitting on the toilet peeing—that's when I have my most contemplative moments."

Thomas Crapper, Closet Genius

Reginald Reynolds said that the kindliest epitaph for the Victorians would have to be "They Attended To Plumbing." How appropriate then that Thomas Crapper, the most inventive plumber of the era, possibly of any era, was born in 1837, the very year Queen Victoria took the throne. The developments Crapper wrought during his eventful career, most of which pertain to his own throne, a device now called "the crapper," have changed our world, bringing ease, comfort, and better health to billions.

Crapper was born in the Yorkshire town of Thorne. When he was eleven years old, he walked to London, 165 miles away, to find work. Eleven years old. 165 miles. The energetic lad soon got a job as a plumber's apprentice in Chelsea, the ever-fashionable London borough he worked out of for the duration of his career. London completed its first two sewer mains in 1861, ushering in a boom time for the city's plumbers. In this same year Crapper, now 24 and quite plumbing-knowledgeable for his age, opened up his own business, the Marlboro' Works, located on one of the London's many streets called Marlborough Road.

Other interesting things were going on with London's infrastructure during this time. The Metropolis Water Act of 1872 unified London's eight separate water companies, each of which had had its own set of regulations, and aimed to curb the city's enormous water usage, much of which was caused by inefficient toilets. Back then, many toilets simply had a plug in the bottom of the water tank. A tug on the chain yanked it out temporarily for each flush before letting it fall back into the hole for the tank to refill. One problem with this design was that an imperfect seal let water trickle out constantly, and as the plug aged the seal only worsened. In addition, it was found that some lazy or overly-fastidious people actually tied the chain down, putting the fixture into an environmentally incorrect nonstop flush mode.

To address these concerns, the Board of Trade solicited plans for a "Water Waste Preventer." Crapper and his Marlboro' Works responded by dusting off a design Sir John Harington had come up with nearly 200 years earlier and then building, testing, and refining until the result, the first modern flush toilet, could neatly flush away such

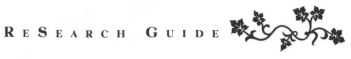

test materials as apples, sponges, cotton, grease, and folded-paper air balloons. On many dramatic occasions the crew would gather around the newest prototype and watch in anticipation as the designated chain puller put the works into motion. During one successful trial, an enthusiastic employee grabbed the cap off an apprentice's head and cast it into the swirling bowl with the cry, "It works!" On another, less fortunate occasion, the intake valve from the large overhead water tank came loose and everyone present got doused with a powerful spray.

In Crapper's design, initiating a flush moves enough water up into a siphon tube to start a flow that empties the contents of the tank into the bowl below at high speed. The bowl goes down to a gooseneck trap which prevents sewer gases from coming up into the room and causes the bowl itself to empty by siphonic action when the deluge of the flush suddenly raises its water level high enough to fill the gooseneck's upper curve. The tank above has a float which shuts off water refilling it once it reaches the proper level. These three elements, the keys to Crapper's design, remain unchanged in today's flush toilets. The only difference from the user standpoint is that back then you pulled a chain, whereas now you push a lever which pulls a chain.

From the Marlboro' Works' first "wash-down closet" on, Crapper's teeming mind produced innovation after innovation and his genius and hard work earned him and his company great success, eventually including a royal appointment as "Sanitary Engineers to His Majesty." The Marlboro' Works' building proudly displayed a 4'x6' crest that signified the appointment.

In 1863, Crapper patented the self-rising seat, which counterweights lifted out of the way between uses. Institutions bought it, but it wasn't popular in homes, partly because elderly users objected to its slapping their bottoms if they didn't precisely coordinate sitting down with letting go of the seat. The product was discontinued in the 1940's.

In 1888, Crapper came out with the cantilever toilet, in which the bowl attached directly to the wall and the wall concealed all the plumbing. He marketed the cantilever not for the sleek designer bathrooms we see them in today, but for prisons and mental institutions where he thought staffs would prefer not to have such hardware as heavy brass chains and metal rods with hollow brass balls on the ends within easy grasp of the toilets' regular users.

In 1891, Crapper patented the Seat Action Automatic Flush—the ultimate in convenience. Simply standing back up activated the flush mechanism. This model never caught on, however, in part because it cost more and people hesitated to splurge on toilets. Also, many people stand to wipe themselves; to clear the bowl of a Seat Action Automatic, these people would have to sit and stand again once their job was completed. This invention of Crapper's suggests that he himself preferred to remain seated throughout his defecation routine, and perhaps assumed that all others did the same.

Crapper also invented silencers to cut down on flush noise, footplate flushers for urinals, and a cistern that flushed urinals at regular intervals without a timer. Another invention of his, the Trough Closet, went through an interesting revision. Schools using the Trough found that mischievous boys would light crumpled pieces of paper and float them "downstream" from the Trough's high end, burning the bottoms of any unfortunate boys seated on the fixture. Crapper soon responded with the Improved Trough Closet, whose more compartmented design prevented such shenanigans.

His need-directed ingenuity even extended outside the bathroom. Soon after an employee of his fell down some stairs, he invented a new type of stair treads.

In 1885, Crapper was in his late forties and his inventiveness may have been at its peak. During this year, the Marlboro' Works and the Twyford company came out with the Unitas, the first "pedestal closet." Until this time, toilets were modestly but unhygienically boxed, a carryover from when they were portable furnishings that simply covered and provided ventilated seating over chamberpots. The Unitas changed all this, bringing the porcelain fixture out into the open for the first time. This superior design soon took over, and as a result, the porcelain lower part, the "pan," became a visible piece of furniture in its own right.

In the Unitas collaboration, the Marlboro' Works manufactured the tank and flush mechanism, where all the moving parts resided, and Twyford, still a leading manufacturer of toilets in Britain today, produced the pan. The Victorian taste for ornament soon had Twyford producing elaborate pans with all sorts of themes. Fixtures sported bas-relief and flat representations of dolphins, lions, flowers, architectural features, and other ornaments, and were known by such names as Niagara, Alerto, Aeneas, Marlboro, Sloane, Cascade, and Pluvius. Other companies got into the act, resulting in scores of different models from which the family could choose in order to make its own decorative statement. A family living near Windsor castle, for example, might select the Windsor, which had a castle motif and featured a picture of Windsor Castle right inside the bowl.

The origin of the Twyford company is interesting in itself. The special type of pottery they started out manufacturing was originally developed by two brothers from Holland who set up a factory in 1690 in Staffordshire, an area known for its good clay. To keep the details of their manufacturing process secret, the brothers made it a policy to employ from the local community only the mentally weak. The two founders of Twyford, Josiah Twyford and John Astbury, pretended to be imbeciles in order to get jobs at the factory. Hired on, they continued with their act and were patiently and repeatedly shown each manufacturing station wherever their unskilled efforts were needed. Two years later, having learned the whole process, they quit the Dutch company, founded their own firm, and started to produce the same pottery at a lower cost. The competition soon drove the Dutch company away, and Twyford's was born.

Another triumph concurrent with the Unitas introduction was Crapper's commission, as His Majesty's Sanitation Engineer, to renovate the plumbing of Sandringham House, a royal estate with a mansion and formal gardens. Here Crapper and the Marlboro' Works took elegance to new heights with amenities such as velvet upholstered armchair toilet enclosures and, for the Queen's bathroom, three separate marble washbasins labeled, in order of descending size, "HEAD & FACE ONLY," "HANDS," AND "TEETH."

The 1880's also brought Thomas Crapper some misfortune. River and ditch dumping and overflowing cesspools made London a breeding ground for typhoid and smallpox, and plumbers were especially susceptible. In 1887, Crapper came down with smallpox. Fortunately he survived and carried on with his work.

Crapper's first great love was his work, but in 1867 he did get married to a woman named Maria Green. Later, as the Marlboro' Works grew, Crapper brought a stern, religious, no-nonsense type named Robert Wharam into the company to run the business side and allow him to concentrate on research and development. Thomas and Maria had no sons, and although Thomas tried to get his nephews involved in the business, none of them worked out. So when Crapper retired he somewhat reluctantly passed the Marlboro' Works over to Wharam. Wife Maria died in 1902 and Crapper himself died in 1910.

It was several years after his death, during World War I, that slang usage gave Crapper some of the honor he deserves. American soldiers stationed in England, many of them farm boys unfamiliar with indoor plumbing, read the "T. Crapper Chelsea" enameled inscription on the lips of the bowls and started calling the contraptions "the crapper." They brought this usage back to the United States, where it remains. Interestingly, although the word "crap" had "feces" as one of its meanings long before Crapper was born, it was originally etymologically unrelated to American slang's "crapper."

Thomas Crapper rests in Elmers End cemetery, not far from the grave of another widely respected and loved Englishman, cricket hero W. G. Grace. Many visitors enjoy the poetry of their juxtaposition. There they are: work and play, industry and sport, brains and brawn, two sides of the same British coin.

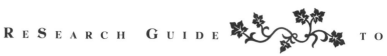

Needless to say, Thomas Crapper was a Mason. *Note: The source for this chapter is Wallace Reyburn's* Flushed With Pride: The Story of Thomas Crapper *(1969). I've seen many references to Crapper published since Flushed With Pride, but I've yet to find a mention pre-dating Reyburn's book. In his review of the book for* Newsweek, *Harry Waters writes, "Although the book has the ring of a classic hoax, Reyburn presents ample evidence that the man not only lived, but made a lasting contribution to mankind's comfort." But until I see a pre-1969 Crapper reference, I'll wonder if Reyburn's evidence isn't just a little* too *ample.*

Excrement in Psychoanalysis

The first few decades of this century were a great time for excrement. Changing morals and the birth of psychoanalysis meant that for the first time, intellectuals could analyze, discuss, and write papers about doo and pee under the banner of Science, and have it therefore be perfectly acceptable. Their understandable glee fueled a period of intense intellectual ferment which elevated lowly feces to the honorable position of Unconscious Symbol for a shitload of important things such as money, genitalia, art, gifts, babies, death, disorder, and foreign elements. Diapering and toilet training, formerly mere chores, became events which profoundly shape the individual's personality and which many debilitating neuroses find their roots in. The scatological legends and practices of various cultures took on a whole new importance with underlying psychological significance. And people's individual scatological rituals and eccentricities became windows into their psyches. In the intellectual arena, feces were suddenly hot shit.

As a result, the pioneers of psychoanalysis, Freud and his circle, produced and left to the field a mountain of thought regarding excrement (feces in particular) including symbolic meanings, how our early experiences cement these meanings, and how our adult behavior is also guided by these experiences. More recently, others, such as Norman O. Brown and Alan Dundes, have expanded on the most important legacy from this body of thought, the concept of the Anal Personality, to explain the illnesses and behaviors of our society as a whole.

A list of all the meanings attributed to shit-as-symbol includes money, genitals, art, babies, gifts, poison, foreigners, and sex. Before exploring the bases for the meanings, here are fuller discussions of the meanings themselves:

Money

Of all the things feces stands for in traditional Freudian psychoanalysis, the best known is probably money (or, equivalently, gold). The link was first presented by Freud in 1908 in "Character and Anal Erotism," the ground-breaking, shocking paper which first described what we now all know as "anal retentive" or "anal" personality characteristics. Drawing on his clinical experience and corroborating with themes from folklore and idiomatic language, Freud explained that children who derive pleasure from their stools early in life often sublimate this tendency later into, among other things, an interest in money. Sandor Ferenczi elaborated upon the course of this gradual redirection of interest in 1914 with "The Ontogenesis of the Interest in Money" by tracing the growing anal-erotic child's favorite playthings from feces to mud to sand to pretty pebbles to marbles, buttons, and other collectibles, and finally, to money itself.

Some of the cultural references Freud and others point to demonstrate the connection are the traditional German *Ducatenscheisser* character, a little man who passes large coins from his anus, depicted most often in little sculptured children's candies, and folk tales such as The Goose That Laid the Golden Egg (note that geese have a cloaca, a single opening for urination, defecation, and reproduction), Rumpelstiltskin, King Midas, and others which indirectly make a connection between gold and excrement or worthless material. They also note that the expression "filthy rich," which has equivalents in other languages, makes the same association. Freud points out that ancient Babylonian and Asian mythologies, which have made their way into much popular legend, both assert that gold is the feces of Hell.

Genitals

Freud associates the penis with the 'column of feces' (the phrase appears in several places in Freud's works) in the lower intestine, and in one study, he connects the childhood constipation of his patient, the "Wolf Man," with fear of castration, fear of becoming separated from his genitals. The unconscious, Freud argues, views feces, male genitalia, and babies in the same way, as objects which can detach from the body. Lawrence Kubie proposes that the irrational fantasy we have that the human body is a "dirt factory" results in the view that women, because they possess an "extra" orifice, are dirtier than men. This vagina-dirt association, he argues, partially explains why women are traditionally more concerned with beautifying and perfuming themselves than men are; it is felt that they have to compensate for being inherently dirtier.

Freud's Wolf Man deserves further discussion. Freud's longest case history, "From the History of an Infantile Neurosis," describes Wolf Man as a wealthy young Russian who could only feel at one with the world after taking enemas administered by one of his attendants. Wolf Man took enemas often, reenacting sexual congress and birth, Freud felt, with the attendant playing the father, Wolf Man himself playing the mother, and the stool resulting from the enema acting as the baby. This reenactment recalled the "primal scene" of the case, a scarring experience in which Wolf Man, as a very small child, walked in on his parents as they were having sexual intercourse "doggie style" (which led to the subsequent fear of dogs and wolves that gave Wolf Man his name in the literature), panicked, cried out, and soiled his pants, interrupting his parents' congress. This event messed up Wolf Man emotionally as well as physically, and one moral of the case, the same as the one in Sue Miller's *The Good Mother*, is clear: don't bone in front of the kid.

Art

I didn't find any feces-as-art discussions in the early psychological literature, but the association was made by artists themselves. In 1918, for example, the political cartoonist George Grosz participated in a protest in which he feigned excretion in front of a painting and declared "Art is shit!" Dali, Dubuffet, Picasso, and DeChirico have all written of art as an extension of defecation. And in one of the best-known rebellious artistic statements of this century, Marcel Duchamp submitted a urinal as sculpture, at the New York Independents' Exhibition in 1917.

Baby

In Freud, the unconscious views babies, like penises, as detachable excrements. Wolf Man, for example, lived for the experience of "giving birth" to a stool after an enema. Freud also notes that young children often view birth as a special sort of defecation. This ties in with the many myths and folk tales in which gods create people through defecation, reflecting men's universal envy of women's procreative ability.

Gift

Freud (again) writes that feces are an infant's first gift to others. Producing them shows compliance with the parents while withholding shows disobedience. Infants never defecate in the arms of strangers, he explains; they only soil the ones they love. The "gift" meaning of feces is the earliest; only later in life does the child refine this original meaning to include "baby," "money," etc.

Poison/Weapon

Melanie Klein explains that when parents encourage elimination and warn children that they'll become sick if they don't defecate, the children

start to view feces as a destructive poison which can harm others as well as the self.

Foreigner/Outcast

Lawrence Kubie calls the notion that the body is essentially a dirt factory "the dirt fantasy" and discusses how this fantasy contributes to prejudice and nationalism. Any representative of a strange group is called "a dirty ____" and groups such as Africans and Jews are often viewed as contaminants to society. Kubie goes on to explain part of white prejudice against darker peoples as an extension of the dirt fantasy which holds that skin color comes from deep within the body just as excrement does, and that the two are related. More recently, Alan Dundes shows how anal personality aspects of German national character came out during the Holocaust, as evidenced by Nazi rhetoric's many references to "cleaning up" the country and its gene pool of the excrement that is non-Aryans. (Fortunately, German anality now seems directed against the filth in our environment; however, the Green Party's zealotry about cleaning up sometimes seems no less fervent than was the Nazis'.)

Sex

In the "Scatologic Symbolism" chapter of his *Studies in the Psychology of Sex* (1906), Havelock Ellis writes that excretion is a dynamic symbol for sex itself, sharing with it the pattern of built-up tension and release of stored material.

Ellis also discusses the origins of scatological fetishism: The idealization of love, which often neutralizes the sensitivity of lovers to their partner's excretions, sometimes goes even further, resulting, in extreme cases, in fetishistic arousal at body products alone, separate from the person who produced them. In addition, the excretory organs' proximity to the genitals positively associates the two. Demonstrating this connection, many children first channel their sex impulses into interest in the scatological.

Ellis mentions "renifleurs" (sniffers), men who hang out around women's privies, wait for them to emerge, and then go in to "excite themselves" by the odor. In one case, the man would enhance his masturbation by licking any wet spot he'd find. Similarly, one woman Ellis discusses preferred to stimulate herself while holding a bottle of stale male urine. She claimed she could tell by the smell if urine was from a man or not, and the smell of fermented male urine so excited her that she would often go off to masturbate after passing street urinals. Ellis also mentions an innovation described by de Sade, the "tabouret de verre" of Parisian brothels which enabled patrons to observe prostitutes' defecation at close range from beneath a glass floor.

Miscellaneous

Freud's Wolf Man also associated feces with God. In fact every time he saw three heaps of horse dung on the road, he automatically thought of the Holy Trinity. For the anal personality, feces means disorder and chaos. Feces can also mean mortality, or at least remind us of it and of the ultimate equality mortality means. In more of a physiological association than a symbol, we link defecation to fright because extreme fright can lead to loss of bowel control, as when Wolf Man was "scared shitless" by seeing his parents copulating. And, finally, a fictional letter from Freud in *National Lampoon* implied that Freud proposed that feces and defecation symbolize work (as opposed to farts, which are "just for fun"). Freud's writings do not support this, but I think it's a good interpretation anyway.

So where did all these meanings come from? How did excrement come to signify so much? The early psychoanalysts point to the importance of diapering and toilet training during the early, formative years of a personality. To the infant, diapering is one of the few constants in a world of variables, regularly providing parental contact, caring, and attention, much like feeding. Toilet training rips this away from the child and lays on an unprecedented new burden of responsibility. Suddenly they're asked to become aware of and control a formerly automatic part of themselves, a totally unanticipated, unfamiliar, and difficult task, and succeed with it at risk of losing parental and societal acceptance. The shock of coming to terms with and accepting this first great burden echoes through the rest of the individual's lifetime.

Another reason traditional psychoanalysis attributes so much importance to toilet training is that the culture that surrounded Freud and his group emphasized it unusually heavily. At the beginning of this century, mothers (fathers had other responsibilities) were taught to commence toilet training as early as possible, to cut down on the drudgery of hand-washing diapers, and, more significantly, to instill early on a sense of order, cleanliness, and respect for authority. Starting as early as one month, they would set aside frequent blocks of time to hold the child over a pot or even strap them down and probe their rectum with soap sticks or glass or porcelain rods until they passed a stool. A rigid toilet regimen was seen as necessary to physical and mental health, and mothers who couldn't toilet train their small infants, which was all of them, were told they were failures.

We have since learned that the nerves used in excretory control cannot carry conscious impulses until the twentieth month, when they've acquired their full myelin sheaths, so until children are newly two, their central nervous systems render them literally incapable of "holding it" no matter what their intentions might be. All the old exercises with soap sticks, straps and regulated potty hours would sometimes by chance coincide with the child's elimination, but it taught the child nothing, and the inevitable "accidents" and the resulting scoldings or even beatings turned toilet training into a years-long battleground between parent and child which, like any other issue turned into a power struggle and blown way out of proportion, did indeed have profound effects on the child's psyche.

Our culture still carries some of that "the earlier the better" message that traumatized so many of Freud's patients. In *Life Is Like A Chicken-Coop Ladder*, folklorist Alan Dundes notes that while most primitive societies typically toilet train at around 24 months, Americans often begin at 18

months and some Germans try it as early as five months, believing that the child should be "housebroken" by one year. But even these timetables aren't as extreme as the ones popular in Freud's day, thanks to washing machines, disposable diapers and diaper services, scientific knowledge, and a little more sense. Nevertheless, other cultures are baffled by Western anthropologists' questions about how they deal with the "problem" of toilet training. For societies that don't worry about it, children learn when they're ready and there is no problem.

Professor Dundes also points to another custom which might cause, or at least evidence, the Teutonic propensity for anality Freud generalized from. The custom is that of swaddling infants in layers of cloth, which prevents them from moving freely and puts them in constant contact with their own excrement for fairly long periods of time. These early experiences of being bound up and both subjected to and protected by a layer of human waste, Dundes submits, might also contribute to the Germans' complex ambivalence toward matters scatological.

Freud suggests yet another origin of our feelings toward excrement, coming not from individual development but from our evolution. As our ancestors adopted an upright posture, sight became more important and smell atrophied, changing our attitude toward excrement. Kubie counters that many cultures seem not to have lost their olfactory acuity, and suggests that while smell may have lost importance in our rational analysis, it could simultaneously have gained importance in close-range emotional judgments such as those associated with eating and sex.

Given all these attitudes we have about excrement and how they may have originated, the question becomes, how do we behave as a result? In our culture, for reasons going way back, we deny excrement and conspire with others to ignore our connection to it. In the individual, this cultural context can foster development of the anal personality, the personality type already mentioned as having a special interest in money. Anal personalities start out, according to Freud, as chil-

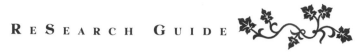

dren who retain their feces intentionally to experience the pleasure of a full colon (many have since questioned Freud on this) because they naturally have a greater-than-average fondness for stimulation of the anal region. Our cleanliness-oriented society discourages this sensual tendency, so these children are forced to strike their first bargain with society: cleanliness for love. They sublimate their scatophilic inclinations into an interest in feces substitutes, money being the most advanced, and begin a lifelong battle against their forbidden inclinations that results in a fascination with order and cleanliness. So natural anal erotics in our culture become orderly, parsimonious and obstinate, the characteristics Freud uses to describe the "anal personality." Freud bolsters his argument by mentioning that he has not seen these three defining traits in those homosexuals who never suppressed their anal erotic tendencies in the first place.

More recently, Norman O. Brown in *Life Against Death* (1959) suggests that anal personality traits not only characterize individuals in our society, but also characterize the society as a whole. He argues, drawing support from sources as diverse as Marx and Keynes, that many of our social ills stem from the essentially anal characters of Capitalism and Scientific Rationality. In their pure form, these systems encourage materialism, mastery over nature, lust for power, irrational desire for luxuries, obsession with death, and alienation. Brown goes on to assert that if we changed our attitudes, if we sought not to rise above our bodies, equating them with excrement and death, but rather accept and enjoy them, then the social problems he discusses, problems ultimately caused by repression, would disappear and humankind would be able to have fun, no longer obsessed by morbid interests in money, power, and status. Science would seek unity with, rather than mastery over, nature and people would abandon uptight, competitive status-seeking and become naturally generous. The technology and social structures we have bought with centuries of paying the high price of anality, could be redirected to create a peaceful, life-loving world.

Brown sounds utopian, but Thomas More himself said some of the same things; in *Utopia*, the chamberpots are made of gold and silver because citizens hold these metals in such contempt.

Similarly, Alan Dundes defends the notion of "national character" by supporting with volumes of evidence the idea that German culture has a strong, deeply rooted anal personality, and that this understanding sheds light on its art, science, and even its Nazi history, demonstrating one very high price of excessive anality.

Holy and Unholy Shit: Excrement In Religion

To Western ears, Religion and Scatology sound like opposites: sacred and profane, clean and dirty, Good and Evil. We believe that being made in God's image and defecating are somehow incompatible, and this cognitive dissonance, according to Milan Kundera, makes shit a more onerous theological problem than evil. But as John G. Bourke and others have catalogued, most of the world's religions throughout history actually embraced scatology. Referring to pre-Christian times, Bourke writes, "The use of human and animal egestae in religious ceremonial was common all over the world," and his treatise *Scatalogic Rites of All Nations*, first published in 1891, details widespread religious use of excrement in both extinct pagan practices and indigenous religions still active at the time. Bourke's book, most of which consists of reports from other anthropologists and observers, suggests that most of the religions people have observed throughout the ages probably regarded the body's products as closer to sacred than to profane.

Three important exceptions, however, are Judaism, Christianity, and Islam, which, unlike most other religions, demonized excrement. The reasons for this can be found in the Old Testament, the sourcebook all three religions share. The anti-scatological stance that distinguished the Israelites from their fertility cult, idol-worshipping neighbors and rivals during Old Testament times became a characteristic part of Jewish culture, and of the Christian and Moslem cultures that sprung from it, and through these three religions, this attitude has exerted a major influence on the progress of world history. Nevertheless, by the standards of most other religions, the attitudes of Western monotheism toward bodily functions must be considered abnormal.

Many of the world's creation myths, for example, explain that the land, the oceans, and the first people came from urine, feces, and menstrual blood of gods, and many gods have a close association with excrement. The prechristian Mexican goddess Suchiquecal, the mother of the gods, and Ixcuina, or Tlacolquani, the goddess of carnal pleasures, are traditionally depicted eating feces, as is the Australian spirit Gunungdhukya.

Some Hindus atone for sins by eating cow dung or drinking panchakaryam, a mixture of the Five Purifying Substances: milk, ghee (clarified butter), curd, dung, and urine, all from the cow. Another use of the number five in Hinduism comes up in the Five Meritorious Suicides, one of which is covering yourself with cow dung and lighting yourself on fire. Hindus, Hottentots, and Dinkas smear themselves with dung or dung ashes to atone, as did the ancient Greeks. The Persians atoned by drinking cow urine. South Australian Aborigines cover themselves with excrement or filthy clothing during mourning, as did the Aztecs. The Hebrews did this as well (Joshua does it in Zechariah 3:3-4), but for them, this sort of ritual was exceptional. According to Bourke, dung and urine have been used in funeral ceremonies on every continent.

Religions don't just use excrement for solemn occasions of lustration and mourning, either. Often, they're used for good luck and for happy occasions such as weddings and festivals. Pious Hindus never pass a urinating cow without catching a few drops to sip for good luck. Tibetan Buddhist followers of the Dalai Lama attribute beneficial properties to the living religious leader's feces, which is dried, powdered, and sold for use as a lucky food condiment, as snuff, as a medi-

cine, and to put in amulets. (In 1889, Bourke procured of some of this sacred dung and, with the help of the Surgeon General, had it chemically analyzed. They found nothing remarkable.)

Bourke lists many Siberian, Eskimo, and Native American cultures which hold what he calls "ur-orgies," religious or quasi-religious celebrations which employ urine. The best-described is the Urine Dance of the Zuñi, an elaborate, frenzied rite with dancers, clowns, music, and a mock sermon in which participants produce and drink large quantities of urine and eat small pieces of corn husks, rags, feces, and other indigestibles. The Zuñi medicine men organize these rites to inure the participants' stomachs to a wide range of foods, giving the ceremony a very practical basis.

But another reason urine drinking shows up in religious rituals has to do with a special property of the fly agaric mushroom (Amanita Muscaria), a hallucinogen that has been employed for religious ceremonial in Siberia and India since prehistoric times.

Active ingredients in the fly agaric mushroom excite the kidneys and can induce vomiting, and its main hallucinogenic component, muscimole, passes through the body unchanged. This set of properties has led many cultures to develop ways of recycling the drug. The most common is simply for participants to drink one another's urine, passing bowls around for the duration of the event. By this method, a single mushroom can help several people "see god" for an entire week. Another method, less common, has one man (by all accounts, only men participate in these rituals) fast for some time and then gorge himself on the mushrooms. He vomits and re-eats the semidigested mushroom concoction several times, after which it is served to the other worshippers, who supplement it with the man's urine. One writer observes that in Yakutsk, when a thoughtful participant in these quasi-religious mushroom orgies first throws up, he does so into a bowl of water. The bowl is then set aside to cool, after which time his family can enjoy a meal of the "rich, floating vomit" that results.

Australia does not naturally grow the fly agaric

mushroom, but the aboriginals in Queensland have found that the nuts of a particular species of pine that grows near Darlington become psychoactive after fermenting in human urine. The men urinate into large clay pans in the ground, wherein they steep the seeds to prepare them.

Meanwhile, there's a quieter side to the scatological dictates of many religions, one that is concerned with routine, daily excretory behaviors. One of the most involved is the toilet ritual of the pious Hindu. Before defecating, he offers the hari-smarana, a prayer to Vishnu that ends with all of Vishnu's thousand names. During defecation, preferably before sunrise, he has to hang his triple cord over his left ear, cover his head with his loin-cloth, stoop as low as possible, avoid looking at the sun, the moon, the stars, fire, a Brahmin, a temple, an icon, or a sacred tree such as a banyan, and keep perfect silence. He must not linger or look behind himself upon rising, and he must do this all within bowshot of his home but away from any river, pond, well, public thoroughfare, plowed field, sacred tree, and light-colored soil. Meanwhile, Hindu yogis are known for their feats of self-control and discipline, one of which is the trained yogi's ability to draw water into his rectum with the sphincter muscles alone, enabling him to self-administer an enema by simply sitting in water. Many yogis also routinely drink their own urine, as is recommended by the Vedas.

But the early Israelites' views of excrement in religious observance, the radical, world altering attitude found in the Old Testament and with us still today, came from their reactions against the religions prevalent in the area at the time. Regarding excrement, these ancient Middle-Eastern religions were as scatologically permissive as any others, if not more so. Like polytheistic religions elsewhere, they worshipped a pantheon of individual gods who watched over different aspects of the mysterious and interrelated phenomena of the universe, including fertility, bodily functions, agriculture, seasons, life, and death.

The Old Testament often refers to one of these gods, Baal-Peor (also known as Baal, Baal of Peor, Bel-Phegor, Baal-Phegor, and Baal-zebub

the god of Ekron), as an idol worshipped by Canaanites, Syrians, Moabites, delinquent Israelites, and others. Most of what we know of the worship of Baal-Peor comes to us from historical accounts critical of paganism, but Baal-Peor seems to have been a "dung god" associated both with the gut, flatulence, and other bodily adjuncts to feces, and with the agricultural fertility linked to dung. Because polytheistic religions typically match sacrificial materials to the gods they're appeasing, Bourke explains, adherents would logically sacrifice flatus and feces to Baal-Peor to cure intestinal troubles or to help fertilized crops grow, just as they would sacrifice fish to the god of the seas to ensure a good catch. Bourke links Baal-Peor backwards to Le Pet, an ancient Egyptian god associated with flatulence, depicted as a small child with a swelled paunch, and forward in time to Crepitus, the Roman god of flatulence and sanitary conveniences.

Many old reports assert that worshipping Baal-Peor did involve making scatological sacrifices of some sort before an altar. By some accounts, this merely meant "sacrificing" a fart. Others explain that adherents bared their bottoms and defecated before the altar at the idol's mouth, which was in the likeness of an anus. Yet another account says that the worshipper would offer the idol tears, earwax, "pus from the nose," saliva, and urine as well as feces. Psalms 106:28 claims that human sacrifices were offered to Baal-Peor, after which the sacrifices were eaten. If this is true, then the sacrifice of scatological materials may have come later, as a symbol of human sacrifice.

The monotheism of the Israelites was a radical departure from the religions that surrounded them, and much of Judaism grows out of enforcing this separation. In the Old Testament, nothing raised God's ire more than when He saw His chosen people worshipping "detestable idols" (Deuteronomy 29:16) or "dungy gods" such as Baal-Peor. Rejecting the gods surrounding peoples worshipped was so central that it was codified as the first two of the sacrosanct Ten Commandments: "I am the Lord thy God..." and "Thou shalt have no other gods before Me..."

Numbers 25 tells a characteristic story. During the Israelites' residence in a land called "Shittim," (the Bible intends no pun) God sees them worshipping Baal-Peor. God complains to Moses, and Moses demands that these Baal-worshippers be slain. An Israelite man presents a Midianitish woman as a suspect, and then another Israelite, Phinehas, flies into a rage and runs both of them through with his spear. In typical Old Testament fashion, God is pleased by this murderous zeal, so he spares the Israelites from a plague, makes a covenant of peace and everlasting priesthood with Phinehas and his descendants, and commands Moses to tell the Israelites to harass and smite the Baal-worshipping Midianites.

To clearly distinguish itself from Baal-worship and other forms of idolatry, which were scatological, Judaism needed to rebel and establish itself as strongly anti-scatological. This it did, as can be seen in the Old Testament.

The Old Testament mentions excrement disparagingly in many places. One image is that of the indignity of the dead being left on the ground, unburied and unremembered, like dung on the field (Second Kings 9:37, Jeremiah 8:2, 9:21, 16:4, 25:33, Job 20:7). In Malachi 2:3, God promises to spread dung on the faces of priests who do not glorify His name.

The Old Testament has several references to coprophagy as well. In Ezekiel 4:12-16, God commands Ezekiel to eat bread baked with human excrement while laying siege to Jerusalem. After Ezekiel then pleads that he has never eaten anything unclean, God tells him he may use cow dung as a substitute. A few commentators explain that the dung is just meant to be the cooking fuel.

In Second Kings 18:26 and Isaiah 36:12, a messenger from the conquering king of Assyria, threatening to destroy Jerusalem if they don't submit to Assyrian rule, insults the Jews by suggesting that they drink their own urine and eat their own dung. Hezekiah, the local king, refuses to surrender, but he does pray to God, and God answers by killing over five thousand Assyrian soldiers one night, soon afterwards causing the King of Assyria to leave the country for a while,

only to return to assassination by his own sons.

More scatological references are in the Old Testament's euphemistic usage of "to cover one's feet" for "to defecate." In I Samuel 24:4 Saul ducks into a cave to "cover his feet" in privacy, only to find rival David and his men in there. Judges 3:20-26 tells how Ehud murdered King Eglon while Eglon was "covering his feet" in the privy, then locks him in there and escapes.

The euphemism makes more sense in light of the commandment in Deuteronomy 23:12-14, which prescribes that when you are in camp against your enemies, you must carry a paddle around with you and use it to bury your excrement, presumably to hide any trace of your presence. Early stealth technology such as this gave the Israelites the military prowess that led to many long-shot victories chronicled in the Old Testament. Interpreters have since taken this commandment to mean that you should always bury your excrement, seeing it as one of the Bible's many general health measures, but the original context specifically refers to the military situation alone.

The only positive, "fun" scatological references I found in the Old Testament are Psalms 78:66 and Proverbs 17:14. The psalm describes the Lord waking up as if with a hangover and smiting his enemies "backwards," suggesting a powerful morning beer fart. Versions of the proverb vary, but in the 1917 translation from the Masoretic Text, it warns that getting into an argument is like urinating: once you start, it's difficult to stop.

Continuing in the cleanliness-is-next-to-godliness tradition, Rabbi Simeon ben Eleasar in the Talmud likens the human body to a large palace with a tannery pipe leading through it and emptying at its doorway, ruining its appeal. More pointedly, tradition has it that Adam and Eve did not defecate until their exile, nor did the Israelites during their 40 years of wandering in the desert following the Exodus, the reason being that the manna they ate, perfect food that dropped down from Heaven, generated no feces (this illustrates the misconception that feces is "used food" and nothing else). Another tradition names a mythical hell-like place "Gehenna" after the sew-

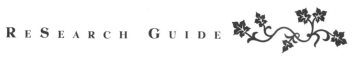

age ditch below Jerusalem's dung gate, the one gate sewage was allowed to pass through. A Christian tradition has it that residents of Heaven do not excrete, excretion being an unpleasant task mortals must endure while on Earth.

Pious Jews are forbidden from praying or studying Torah while they feel the urge to defecate. During defecation, they avoid facing toward or away from Jerusalem and do their best to clear their minds of both holy matters and sinful thoughts.

As a rule, the gods of vanquished or superseded religions become the devils of the religions that take their place, so as Judaism and the religions it spawned spread, Baal-Peor became a devil and all scatological worship became devil worship. The scatological became unholy, a realm of evil, and deriving any pleasure from elimination became sinful. Jews carried this attitude with them as they dispersed, and then Christianity and Islam, rooted in Judaism, picked it up and spread it much further, so that by today, most of the world's population has been exposed to and has to varying degrees adopted Western monotheism's view that excrement is evil. Rooted in the religious differences of rival tribes in the Middle East thousands of years ago, this view has outlasted and outgrown its original purpose and has shaped entire cultures and world events with an impact psychologists and anthropologists have only relatively recently begun to explain.

But this is jumping ahead. All the way up until the era of Constantine the Great (288?-337), the first Christian Emperor, the leading religions in the West were earthy and polytheistic. Crepitus, the Roman god of flatulence and sanitary conveniences, was joined in the Pantheon by, among others, Cloacina, goddess of sewers and privies, Stercutius, Saturn's persona as the inventor of agriculture, and Stercus, the divine inventor of manuring. Similar from the Christian perspective were other Roman gods such as Priapus, god of male procreative power, who was always depicted with an exaggerated erection.

When Christianity spread through Europe, a long battle began. Following the anti-Baal tradi-tion, the Church demonized traditional folk fertility rites involving excrement or menstrual fluid. The new Christian order was also threatened by Paganism's empowerment of women, so the Church adopted those popular beliefs it could recast in a Christian mold, yielding the cult of Mary and the special domains of the patron saints, and suppressed by force other forms of worship with witch hunts, inquisitions, and crusades.

Meanwhile, the more intellectual side of the fight continued on its own terms. In 831, a monk named Paschasius Radbert sparked an inevitable controversy when he wrote that the communion host, which according to Christian doctrine becomes Christ's body during the ceremony of the Eucharist, was liable to digestion and all its consequences just like any other food. Many objected to this assertion, but to my knowledge, no one has tested it by eating only transsubstantiated communion wafers for a whole day to see what happens.

The Church did not authorize early Christian writings that had a scatological tone, such as the First Gospel of the Infancy of Jesus Christ, which tells of miraculous healing properties demonstrated by Christ's soiled swaddling clothes and used bath water. This gospel gives a flavor of the pagan influence on some sects of early Christianity, or at least the early, suppressed, fringe-element Christianity of the Apocrypha.

Much later, but following in the tradition, came Martin Luther's repeated linking of feces and the Devil in his writing and, presumably, his oratory. Luther had an unusually scatological turn of mind. His "epiphany in the tower," the new neural connection that fired in his head and sparked the Reformation, happened to him while he struggled with constipation, a chronic problem of his which he viewed as an inability to escape from the evil within him.

Where scatological worship did survive in Europe was in quasi-religious pagan-holdover festivals such as the Feast of Fools, an annual rite performed until the 18th Century in which participants went naked, cross-dressed, or painted themselves as clowns, took control of a church during high mass, ate sausages at the altar, and then stormed outside to throw excrement from dung carts at the crowd of onlookers. Bourke shows that there's a long tradition in Europe of using sausages to symbolize feces (as Al Jaffee did more recently in a *MAD* cartoon piece on doggie pooper scoopers, reprinted in *MAD Super Special #27*, 1978), and postulates that earlier versions of the Feast of Fools included actual coprophagy. Some historians trace the Feast of Fools back to the Roman Saturnalia festival, a wintertime festival that the church co-opted and converted into Christmas, which would make the scatological Feast of Fools a cousin to the modern day Christmas. Bourke, however, asserts that the origins of the Feast of Fools lie much further back than Roman times, and that the festival is unrelated to Saturnalia.

Recent history provides another example of Christian scatological denial. When a Vatican architect submitted plans for a new administrative building to Pope John the 23rd (1958-63), the visionary Pope looked at the plans and gave the criticism, "They are not angels" (Non sunt angeli). The plans had included no bathrooms!

The diabolization of feces and the more general Judeo-Christian-Islamic denial of the flesh that subsumes it have certainly spread because Christianity and Islam have carried it. But the reverse may also be true as well. The anti-scatological outlook may have likewise contributed strongly to the vigor of the two religions, and the reason why suggests that the outlook has affected history in far more areas than religion alone. Psychology provides the explanation.

Freud describes the "orderly, parsimonious, and obstinate" anal personality as arising out of early repression of the desire to play with feces and seek anal gratification, tendencies which cultures guided by anti-scatological religions strongly discourage. The Old Testament-based religions, then, have the influence of producing large numbers of anal personalities in the populations that adopt them. This is what Erich Fromm, Norman O. Brown and others have suggested; in giving up anal erotism, a culture gains values regarding time, work, money, and personal property, and these characteristically anal-retentive values are what fuel capitalism, industry, and technology, all of which can greatly increase a culture's influence and power. Small wonder, then, that the anti-scatological religions took over so completely. Anality alone didn't fuel these religions' expansions, of course, but it certainly helped.

However, as Fromm and Brown also point out, there's a catch. The engines of progress, life-improving though they may be, stop short of their full potential by remaining mired in an essentially morbid, life-denying outlook. In war and economic policy we value control over human life. Our science has sought domination over nature rather than unity with nature, and we see the morbid effects in our dangerous pollution of the planet. In *Zen and the Art of Motorcycle Maintenance* (1974), Robert M. Pirsig discusses the same "bargain" when he writes that his protagonist:

". . .began to see for the first time the unbelievable magnitude of what man, when he gained power to understand and rule the world in terms of dialectic truths, had lost. He had built empires of scientific capability to manipulate the phenomena of nature into enormous manifestations of his own dreams of power and wealth—but for this he had exchanged an empire of understanding of equal magnitude: an understanding of what it is to be a part of the world, and not an enemy of it."

Fortunately, many people are responding to recent political events and scientific findings with much more of a cooperative, life-affirming outlook and seem willing to throw over antique prejudices that now threaten our survival. The life-denying, anti-scatological stance that Western religions broadcast has given us some powerful tools and social structures which we can now, if we decide to, redirect toward more positive goals.

Filth Pharmacy: Excreta In Medicine

When we think of how doctors use excrement

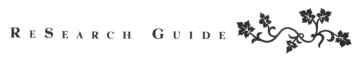

today, we think of stool samples, urine tests, and other diagnostics. Until relatively recently, however, doctors used excrement in treatment as well, and before the late 18th Century's sanitary revolution and Pasteur and Koch's early 19th Century discoveries demonstrated the medical value of cleaning and deodorizing, physicians followed and contributed to the long and worthy tradition of excrement cures known as Filth Pharmacy, or *Dreck Apotheke*, its German name. Today, many argue that by hastily and completely abandoning this millennia-old tradition, the medical establishment may have thrown the baby out with the bathwater.

Once, all the world's doctors, shamans, witches, medicine men, and other types of health care providers relied heavily on remedies made of the body products of people and animals. A fair listing limited just to cures used in Europe would fill hundreds of pages. Pioneering Chemist and Physicist Robert Boyle said that the medical virtues of human urine alone, as a tonic, salve, etc. could fill a volume (such a volume was actually published in 1692, the year after Boyle's death, under the name "B."—coincidence?). Uneducated people believed in Filth Pharmacy folk remedies, but so did the best doctors, and a list of its well-known adherents reads like a Who's Who of Early Medicine: Hippocrates, Xenocrates, Pliny, Galen, Avicenna, Paracelsus, Van Helmont, etc. During the hundred years before the start of the sanitary revolution, a rash of medical texts compiling Filth Pharmacy remedies were published by doctors who distilled millennia of experimentation, corroboration, and belief into single references.

Modern science would undoubtedly refute much of this discarded prophylaxis, but if some of it contains some truth, then as Dr. Theodor Roseberry argues in *Life On Man* (1969), science can now help find this truth and disregard the rest. Roseberry points out that even today we sometimes prescribe drugs on the basis of "symptomatic empiricism" alone, the same trial and error process that evolved Filth Pharmacy in the first place. Scientists would do well to analyze

the chemistries of these initially off-putting folk remedies to find out which of their components, if any, can actually heal. They may uncover some real surprises, as have been found with many curative-agent-containing vegetables and fungi that other branches of folk medicine prescribe. Without good reason, we shouldn't ignore an entire branch of experience in healing because of a relatively new set of cultural distastes.

A cure-by-cure list of Filth Pharmacy remedies would probably only interest people who are experimenting or looking for something in particular. For the rest of us, the following description should paint a general picture: Filth Pharmacy cures use virtually any kind of excrement you can name (badger dung, wild boar urine, crocodile dung, dung of milk-feeding lambs, the urine of an undefiled boy, hare urine, hawk dung, human feces, etc.), prescribe them in pretty much any manner you can imagine (to ingest, to apply as a lotion or poultice, to fumigate and inhale, to inject, to mix with food and drink and ingest, to reduce to ashes and plug into tooth cavities, to use as an infusion for tea, as a suppository, as snuff, and so on), alone or in various combinations, in order to treat pretty much any ailment you can think of (dysentery, tuberculosis, deafness, dandruff, melancholia, delirium, baldness, snakebite, sore breasts, warts, cancer, insomnia, cataracts, plague, etc.). Some recipes were also used, unsurprisingly, simply to induce vomiting. Medical texts written and used by many of history's greatest doctors contained long lists of these excrement remedies.

One expert in Filth Pharmacy, Rosinus Lentilius, argued in 1694 that human excrements could have no therapeutic value because if they were useful to the body, Nature would not have us void them. Galen also disapproved of using human feces, but for purely "aesthetic" reasons. Lentilius's argument relies on the questionable assumption that our bodies are perfectly efficient. Pliny, reflecting a more common view, wrote, "Peacocks swallow their dung, it is said, as though they envied man the various uses of it."

Medicine also employed other body products

and excreta, as did the once-related field of witchcraft. Hair, nails, saliva, earwax, sweat, menstrual fluid, semen, blood, placentas, cauls, gallstones, kidney stones, and tartar scraped from teeth were burned, distilled, fed to dogs, made into charms and amulets, sacrificed, used to sprout seeds, powdered and snuffed, manipulated and observed in various ways, and buried at crossroads during the full moon in order to cure disease, ward off evil, exorcise spirits, spark or extinguish feelings of love, predict the sex of infants, learn the fates of departed relatives' souls, and so on.

When we imagine humanity's earlier attitude towards body products, we can understand how Filth Pharmacy arose. Long ago, body products held a mysterious place between living and inanimate, and we treasured, feared, and revered them for their usefulness in mysterious areas such as fertilizing crops as well as mundane ones like washing cups and bowls. It made sense to use these wondrous substances in and on the body to do good, just as we used them elsewhere. Countless subsequent generations of exploration, experimentation, and debate over this broad and complex set of organic materials began, and a mixture of superstition, wishful thinking, and genuine healing yielded the Filth Pharmacy now recorded in arcane 18th Century medical texts.

One of the greatest practitioners of Filth Pharmacy was the 16th Century doctor Paracelsus, who, showing an early understanding of the sorts of image issues medical professionals still face, gave human feces the code names "Zibethum Occidentalis" and "Oriental Sulphur" and prescribed it under those names for a variety of ailments. More importantly, Paracelsus expanded upon doctors' use of urine and feces in diagnosis-roles they retain ever more usefully today.

The practice of examining excrement dates back a long way. Centuries ago, doctors would taste small amounts of patients' stools, thereby performing a chemical analysis the "natural" way (Grimmelshausen's *Simplicius Simplicissimus* mentions this procedure). They also would inspect the urine's color, churn it and listen to the bubbles, and do other fairly simple things. In one old test, doctors poured urine over sand; if the wet sand attracted insects, the patient had diabetes. Medieval medical texts contained color charts showing different shades of urine and what they revealed. Paracelsus originated what he called the "dissection" of urine, which included distilling it, measuring its specific gravity, precipitating deposits out of it to check them for salt, sulfur, and mercury, and other techniques, all of which provided much more useful information than inspection alone. The belief prevailed that all of human anatomy was somehow represented in the urine. Today we know this isn't far from the truth; the urine contains a chemical record of many of the body's recent activities as well as discarded cells containing its genetic material, and as urine analysis gains precision and sophistication, its power as a non-invasive diagnostic tool increases.

Excretal Customs Worldwide

Before launching into an Other Cultures Do The Darndest Things list in his essay "Of Custom," Montaigne generalizes, "I think that there falls into man's imagination no fantasy so wild that it does not match the example of some public practice," and after recounting various traditions of cannibalism, mutilation, sex, etc., he recaps with "There is nothing that custom will not or cannot do; and with reason Pindar calls her, so I have been told, the queen and empress of the world." The world's body product-related customs, including toilet habits, courtesies, traditions, and even punishments, cover a wide field through which Pindar's queen and empress has cut some divergent and often convoluted paths. Montaigne illustrates by telling of a friend who blew his nose into his hand, common practice in many countries, and wondered what made snot so precious to people that they would wrap it in a special piece of linen and carry it around with them rather than leave it behind like other body products. In Ian Fleming's *You Only Live Twice*, the head of the

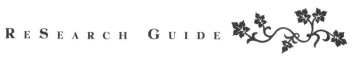
Japan's secret service, Tiger Tanaka, wonders at the same thing. Our handkerchief habits disgust many foreigners, as do our toilet paper habits. The idea of wiping—smearing, really—with a dry piece of paper revolts a large percentage of the Earth's human inhabitants because only something moist, they feel, can effect a real deep-down cleansing. Something moist, like a wet left hand. And we can easily imagine how toting packaged snot around and smearing our feces-besmirched anuses with paper could be considered disgusting. When we look at these customs with new eyes, while retaining familiar values, they *do* seem disgusting.

Our journey through some of the world's scatological customs begins in a logical place: with the excretory acts themselves, where main issues are posture, wiping strategy, context, and method of disposal.

Hand-wiping cultures, most of which are in the Middle East, India, and Africa, generally designate the left hand as the wiper, leading to some secondary, related customs. Best known is the tradition of eating and passing food to others with the right hand only. These cultures consider serving someone food with the left hand a serious insult. A European remnant of this left-behind tradition shows up, according to one explanation, in the ancient association of the left hand and left-handedness with evil, reflected in the meaning the English language gave to the Latin word for left: "sinister." The tradition also provides an easy way to broadcast your wealth and ability to retain personal servants; nobility in China and elsewhere who grew long the fingernails of their left hands were exploiting this mechanism.

Except for around the Mediterranean, the West favors a seated posture for defecation. The rest of the world prefers the more natural squat. Feces disposal has spawned other customs. The Biblically-endorsed practice of digging with a stick and burying it was common not only among Jews, but also Turks and native populations in North America, Southeastern Australia, Borneo, and the Marquesas Islands in Polynesia.

Urination posture customs conveniently split cultures into four groups: everyone stands, everyone sits or squats, men stand while women sit or squat, and women stand while men sit or squat. (A little spread-legged experimentation in the shower will convince any skeptical women from our women-sit culture that all four of these categories are possible.) In *Scatalogic Rites of All Nations* (1891), Bourke makes a special study of urination posture. Much of his information is now no longer valid, but he describes the following divisions:

Most European and European-derived cultures are men standing, women sitting, although until the early 1800s, many European women wore long dresses without underwear and could urinate discreetly while standing, if necessary, by straddling a gutter and looking off into the distance for a while. Parisian, Amazon, lower class Italian, and elderly Swiss women also urinated while standing.

Cultures in which women stood and men sat or squatted were the Apaches, Mojaves, ancient Egyptians, aboriginal Australians, ancient Irish, and Maori (New Zealand). Turks all sat, and considered it heresy to urinate while standing. The Angolans and Chinese, on the other hand, all stood, and some high-ranking Chinese men even ducted their urine through hollow, gilded canes. Maori, Bedouin, and Apache men urinated while walking, as did the lazzaroni, the homeless in Naples.

In Greenland and Iceland, people urinated at the dinner table into a chamber pot servants place underneath when bid to. Siberians had a similar custom in which a fashionable lady's servant received her urine by holding a sponge underneath her dress.

Our tour takes us to courtesies. The Chukchi of Siberia and the English and Dutch of Elizabethan times independently practiced the same one: "drinking flapdragons," as the English called it, meaning toasting to someone's health by drinking a draught of urine. For Europeans and Siberians alike this gesture showed gallantry, but the Siberians also used it to cement friendships, with

the newly-sworn allies drinking both their own and each others' urine.

The French had another interesting custom. There, the King or other nobles would bestow a great honor upon favored subjects by giving them an audience while sitting on the toilet. This special favor came to be known as the "French Courtesy" although it dates back to Roman practice during the 1st Century A.D. The ever-ready chaise percée ("pierced chair," the French version of the close stool, a portable seat enclosing a chamberpot) was popular in the French court, providing royalty ample opportunity to extend the French Courtesy at a moment's notice. The practice had its risks, however. In 1589, France's King Henry III was murdered on the chaise percée. One old English formality required that people defecating by a road take their hats in their teeth and fling them back over their heads if any passer-by called the word "reverence" out to them. A roadside defecator who refused to comply might be pushed backwards. Bourke surmises that the practice was originally intended to ward off the stranger's evil eye during a vulnerable moment, and it probably begat the phrase "sir-reverence," short for "save your reverence," once used like "pardon my French" is now, to excuse vulgar language in advance.

For the last scatological formality on our itinerary, we note that that the Sioux and Assiniboines of the Northern Plains swore oaths to each other while holding buffalo chips.

Many scatological traditions, like many other traditions, connect with life's milestones. At birth in France and Scotland, the mother's breasts were washed with a healthy man's urine. Similarly, natives in California and rustic New England nurses would directly feed urine to newborns.

Throughout Europe there is an old custom, probably of pagan origin, of sprinkling the assembly after the wedding with either the bride's bath water or the bride's urine. Another old European custom has the couple urinate through the wedding band shortly after the marriage to ward off bad luck. Medicine men in southern Africa sprinkled their urine on the young couple, while in northern Africa the bride's urine was sprinkled on the guests. In England and Ireland the guests drank the bride's urine, although the present-day English and Irish have substituted shared chalices of wine or whisky. In northeastern Siberia, among the Chukchi, the bride and groom drink each other's urine.

Several traditions connect unwanted children with dungheaps. Ancient Romans left unwanted children on dungheaps, which were actually registered as their birthplaces. English tradition prescribed that mothers of children thought to be changelings leave the children on dunghills and not to pity them.

The male Australian aborigine initiate can look forward to being covered with feces as part of his rite of passage. Similarly, the male American freshman can look forward to being showered with urine and beer as a part of his college fraternity initiation ritual. Some fraternities employ dog feces as well. As with rites of passage in other cultures, young American "pledges" must endure a series of physically demanding ordeals administered by their elders, including beatings, poisonings, and rituals of humiliation, while other elders smoke hemp and observe, offering the initiates no assistance until they have completed their tasks and are ceremoniously admitted into the fold of manhood. (Those who would have us believe that our culture suffers for lack of a male rite of passage need look no further than the local college and the inanities reverently performed there each Fall.)

Each morning, men of the Achuar Jivaro tribe in Peru and Ecuador drink large quantities of a caffeine-laden tea made from *Ilex guayusa*, and then vomit most of it back up, giving them a good jolt to start the day with. *Ilex guayusa* is closely related to mate, or Paraguay tea (*Ilex paraguayensis*).

Young lovers in Elizabethan England would exchange "love apples," peeled apples they prepared by keeping them in their armpits for several days. The partners would then carry the apples around with them and be able to inhale their sweethearts' fragrances at any time.

Several scatological traditions spice up annual

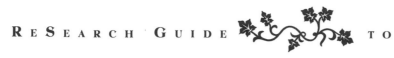
holidays such as the Feast of Fools and other religious and quasi-religious festivals. Harvest festivals also have their traditions of filth. In Germany, farm laborers would play a harvest game in which everyone would cover one of them in dung, wheel him into town in a wheelbarrow, and throw him on the dunghill. During the harvest in Zeeland, Netherlands, a stranger passing by workers digging up madder roots might call out "koortspillers" (a term of reproach) and run. If the workers can catch him, they bring him back, bury him up to his waist while laughing and jeering at him, and defecate in front of his face.

Traditions can also be no more than simple pranks. One old Oxfordshire Mardi Gras custom similar to our trick-or-treating involved groups of boys strolling from house to house singing and demanding eggs and bacon. The boys would frequently stuff the front door keyholes of noncomplying residents' houses with dung.

Another schoolboy custom, this one from 19th Century Philadelphia, demanded that after any audible fart all members of a party of boys would yell "Touch wood!" and run to the nearest treebox. The faster boys would then (of course) beat up on the slower ones.

Europe provides a genuine crime custom, not just a prank: Freud's "grumus merdae," also know as "posting a watchman." In this tradition, which recalls a time when criminals had stronger codes of conduct, burglars would defecate on the floor at the scene of their crime, originally because an ancient superstition held that this would give them a block of time free from interruption. Modern forensic science has increased the riskiness of the practice, but it remains so appealing on so many different levels, that thieves in Edinburgh (and probably elsewhere) do it still. The modern day urban legend about the thief who takes pictures with his vacationing victim's camera of the victim's toothbrush in his rectum gives a modern spin to the same criminal "statement" that the grumus merdae makes.

Crimes usually calls for a trial and sentencing, and many scatological customs take care of these as well. Luandans in Africa relied on a special tea made from "imbando root" which in high enough doses makes people unable to urinate. If the suspect can urinate after drinking some, he's declared innocent. In Sierra Leone they used the opposite approach. Accused poisoners would have to drink a preparation called "red water" and were found guilty if they failed to retain all urine and feces for the next twenty-four hours.

The ducking stool was a popular spectator punishment in England and the U.S. The humiliated criminals would be tied into a chair attached to the end of a levered beam which would be maneuvered to dunk them repeatedly in the town refuse ditch. The English also administered the punishment of forcing prisoners to fast on bread and chicken dung-defiled water.

The Chinese exacted the cruelest scatological penalty however. They enclosed criminals out on the streets in boxes filled with quicklime (which burns when moisture touches it) and put salty foods and water within their reach. The criminals would eventually eat the food out of extreme hunger, then drink the water out of extreme thirst, and burn themselves to death once they urinated any more than just a little bit. This method of punishment adds another entry to the long list of clever and inventive torture and execution methods developed to serve justice and morality.

Bodily Functions in Literature

Aristophanes (448?-380)

Nearly all of Aristophanes' comedies have some scatological humor, but *The Frogs* has more than most. It starts out with a bunch of fart jokes involving Strepsaides and his ungrateful playboy son Pheidippides. Later, Philosophy and Sophistry, "personified" as huge fighting cocks in gold cages, debate the shame of being publicly reamed rectally with a radish. At the end, Pheidippides beats Strepsaides while Strepsaides criticizes him for never helping him to the toilet, when for all those years Strepsaides helped infant Pheidippides to go there whenever he needed to.

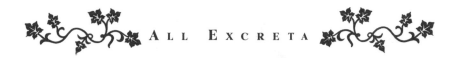

Gaius Valerius Catullus (84?-54)

Number 23 of Catullus's *Poems* discusses how carefree a poor man and his parents are, and suggests that were they better fed, their body products would be that much more burdensome and disgusting. In poem 39, Catullus makes fun of a contemporary, Egnatius, for his constant and often inappropriate smiling, and surmises that he keeps his teeth so white by cleaning them with his own urine.

Dante Alighieri (1265-1321)

In *Inferno*, the river Styx is filthy and slimy, the moat around Dis, the inner part of Hell, smells disgusting, and a foul stench emanates from the inner circles. In the second pocket of the eighth circle, flatterers flounder in a huge lake of shit.

Giovanni Boccaccio (1313-1375)

In the fifth story from the second day of *The Decameron*, Andreuccio, in Naples for the first time, tries to defecate from a plank running between two houses and falls into a shitpile in the alley. In the ninth story from the eighth day, Buffalmacco (of Bruno and Buffalmacco, two wacky troublemakers who appear in several Decameron stories) gets revenge on a doctor by throwing him into a shitpile.

Geoffrey Chaucer (1340?-1400)

Several of the *Canterbury Tales* are scatological, but the strongest is probably the Miller's Tale, a ribald tavern tale of cuckoldry and deceit whose slapstick ending has the main characters farting in each others' faces, burning each others' anuses with hot pokers, and falling down from the rafters. (Some older translations omit the farting, turning the tale into an involved setup with no comprehensible punch line.)

Francois Rabelais (1490?-1553)

Alongside Jonathan Swift, Rabelais is one of the two greatest scatologists in western literature, and, reflecting this, "Rabelaisian" has become a highbrow synonym for "coarse." The best-known scatological passage from *Gargantua* and *Pantagruel* is

Book I, Chapter 13's story of how the five-year-old Gargantua shows early promise by experimenting with a wide variety of objects to wipe himself with before discovering the ideal ass-wipe: the neck of a living goose. Another particularly earthy story is in Book II, Chapter 33: Pantagruel tries to cure his constipation with huge amounts of laxatives, but finally resorts to swallowing teams of workmen encased in copper capsules. Once inside, the workmen leave the capsules, locate the lump of impacted feces, break it up with shovels, cart it away, and then return to the capsules to be vomited back out. The cure is a success.

William Shakespeare (1564-1616)

Shakespeare's references to bodily functions amount to a smattering of jokes and puns scattered throughout his plays, rather than actual situations or subject matters. While he does make plays on the words "water," "wind," etc., Shakespeare's reputation for earthy humor probably comes more from sex jokes than toilet jokes, and is exaggerated even with respect to these. To my knowledge, no Shakespeare play contains more than a handful of dirty jokes (merely an observation, not a criticism).

Hans Jakob Christoffel von Grimmelshausen (1621?-1676)

In *Simplicius Simplicissimus*, the simpleton protagonist farts reekingly while dancing with a high-born woman at a ball and is locked in a dung-filled shed as punishment. There he witnesses a privacy-seeking couple going at it, and soils himself. Later he discusses with a doctor the doctor's diagnostic practice of tasting patient's stools. The novel also contains several episodes of ass-licking and other scatological escapades.

Jonathan Swift (1667-1745)

Swift is widely considered the most scatological of all great writers. His best-known work, *Gulliver's Travels* (or *Travels into Several Remote Nations of the World...by Lemuel Gulliver*, for the hypercorrect), contains many excrement-related passages. In Lilliput, where Gulliver is a giant, he

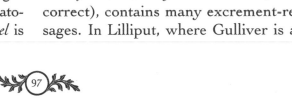

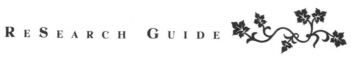

astonishes the Lilliputians after his capture by urinating in front of them, employs two servants with wheelbarrows full-time to dispose of his stools, and saves the burning Lilliputian palace by urinating on it. In Brobdingnag, where he's a midget, he's disgusted by the close-up sights and smells of Brobdingnagian people's skin, lice, blemishes, etc., and is particularly repulsed by watching them eating. He relieves himself in the garden, between two sorrel leaves, and at one point tries to jump over a cow paddy, but lands right in the middle. In Lagado, where the inhabitants are Gulliver's size, Gulliver tours the Grand Academy, where professors and scientists try to convert human excrement back into food, teach mathematics students by feeding them wafers with proofs written on them (which they usually throw up), develop instructions for revealing traitors by examining suspects' stools and toilet habits, and attempt other strange tasks. Arriving in the country of the Houyhnhms, Gulliver first meets the Yahoos when they pelt him with feces. Taken into the care of a family of Houyhnhms, intelligent horses, he learns more about the habits of the filthy Yahoos, including their custom of driving deposed leaders from office by pissing and shitting on them. From the Houynhnms' perspective, Englishman Gulliver sees many parallels between Yahoo culture and his own, and Swift's searing caricature of the human animal has put "yahoo" into the language as a synonym for "boor."

Many of Swift's other writings discuss or allude to bodily functions, including *A Tale of a Tub*, and many poems. His most famous scatological poems, "The Lady's Dressing Room," "Strephon and Chloe," and "Cassinus and Peter," explore the superficial dissonance between romantic attraction and excretion. With humor and insight, Swift concludes that feminine beauty is like the miracle of a flower growing out of muck (an important Zen image as well), and that people should choose their mates for their sense, decency, and friendship rather than beauty and youth.

Tobais Smollett (1721-1771)

In Smollett's last novel, *The Expedition of Humphry Clinker*, Dr. L--n, an 18th Century version of W.S. Burroughs's Dr. Benway, extols the virtues of excrement and strong smells. He himself regularly cheers himself up by inhaling the stirred-up contents of a close-stool, and tells a sickly man he would be happy to drink the liquid that drains from the man's abdomen after it is lanced. Later, the sick man faints from breathing the sweaty stink at a crowded dance. A scene toward the end describes a practical joke played on a gluttonous judge in which he's fed an emetic and a laxative along with a large meal, resulting in a panicked (but spectacular) "double evacuation."

The Marquis de Sade (Donatien-Alphonse-Francois de Sade (1740-1814)

120 Days of Sodom describes a four-month orgy hosted by four wealthy libertines. As well as portraying the violent perversions Sade's work is known for, the novel describes episodes of sexual fetishizing of mucus, saliva, sweat, urine, toe cheese, menstrual blood, miscarriages, vomit, farts, semen, vaginal secretions, and feces. Each of these substances is eagerly consumed by frenzied, pleasure-seeking gentlemen, with feces inspiring the highest levels of connoisseurship. One young financier only eats feces that have been aged for over a week, preferring it moldy. Another man prefers diarrhea, favoring women suffering from indigestion or who have taken laxatives. A landowner keeps a young woman in his home and restricts her to a special diet (low on fat, lots of poultry, and no fish, salted meat, eggs, dairy products, or bread) in order to enhance the flavor of her stools, which he consumes daily. A freethinker takes communion and has four whores shit on the Host while It is still in his mouth.

Johann Wolfgang von Goethe (1749-1832)

In *Götz von Berlichingen*, the doomed rebel knight Götz, surrounded by his enemies and asked to surrender, answers with "Tell your captain. . .he can lick my ass!" The "lick my ass" (leck mich im Arsch) line is roughly the German equivalent of our "fuck you" and "kiss my ass" combined, but with a long literary tradition behind it. Germans politely refer to the line as "the Götz retort," "the Götz quote," "the classical retort," "the well-known reply from Götz von Berlichingen," etc.

Mark Twain (Samuel Clemens, 1835-1910)

In 1876, Twain was visiting friends at their home in Elmira, New York. He was reading Samuel Pepys's diaries, and got such a kick out of them that he decided to write a parody. The result was "1601," subtitled "Conversation As It Was at the Fireside in the Time of the Tudors," an imagined conversation with Queen Elizabeth, Sir Walter Raleigh, William Shakespeare, Sir Francis Bacon, Ben Jonson, and others, during which heavy farting begins to dominate the conversation. The piece drifted around in manuscript form and eventually came into the possession of John Hay, who later served as Teddy Roosevelt's Secretary of State. In 1880, Hay sent it to a publisher friend of his, with a note remarking that, "It was written by Mark Twain in a serious effort to bring back our literature and philosophy to a sober and chaste Elizabethan standard. But the taste of the present day is too corrupt for anything so classic." Since then, taste has remained "too corrupt" and the piece has remained relatively unknown. It has been reprinted a few times, mostly privately or by small presses, and never made it into any of the major Twain anthologies.

Twain also outlined the plot for novel set in Germany's Black Forest, where, Twain noted, residents pile manure in front of their houses as a status symbol. The story focussed on a young woman from a manure-rich family and her three manure-seeking suitors. It ends happily, with the woman's marraige to a man who had recently, by chance, dug into a vast underground pocket of solid manure.

Alfred Jarry (1873-1907)

On a famous night in theater history, 10 December 1896, Jarry's *Ubu Roi* opened at the Theatre de L'Oeuvre in Paris. The play's first word, "merdre" (shit), immediately caused the audience to riot for a full fifteen minutes. Some left, some applauded, some whistled, and in the orchestra, a fistfight broke out. The play, about how Père Ubu (name since adopted by the totally hot rock band) murdered his way to the throne of Poland only to be ousted by his son, contains the word "merdre" in several places. Some critics liked the play, but most did not, one of them beginning his review with, "Despite the late hour, I have just taken a shower." William Butler Yeats's famous comment about upstart Jarry's play was, "After us, the Savage God." Yeats was right; Jarry's "merdre" had changed the theater irrevocably, and Jarry is now considered the founder of avant-garde drama.

Pablo Picasso (1881-1973)

Picasso's only play, *Desire Caught by the Tail*, is a scatological farce about life during wartime.

James Joyce (1882-1941)

In his historic 1933 decision to lift the Federal ban on Ulysses, Judge John M. Woolsey writes that while parts of the book may be "somewhat emetic," the book as a whole is not obscene. Among other bawdy passages, *Ulysses* includes a detailed description of Leopold Bloom's defecating and wiping himself ("Hope it's not too big to bring on piles again. No, just right. So. Ah!"), and ends with a forty-five page punctuationless train of thought from Molly Bloom, in which she realizes that she can arouse her lover by commanding him to "smell rump or lick my shit." Also, in the first few pages of the book, Stephen Dedalus and Buck Mulligan use the expression "the snotgreen sea," playing on *The Odyssey*'s "the wine-dark sea," to help set up the whole "updated Odyssey" angle for the rest of the book.

Jun'ichiro Tanizaki (1886-1965)

In *In Praise of Shadows*, Tanizaki explicates and celebrates the tranquility that the design of the traditional Japanese toilet affords its user.

Erich Maria Remarque (1898-1970)

In *All Quiet On The Western Front*, Remarque asserts that the soldiers' happiest hours are the ones they spend together in the large general la-

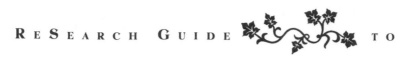

trine, reading, chatting, and playing a game called (appropriately) "skat." He also explains that scatological language is the most direct and honest way for soldiers to express themselves. (Corroborating this, Dan Sabbath, in *End Product: The First Taboo* (1977), writes about a Korean War veteran who, for months after his return, used only the word "shit," conveying his meanings entirely through inflection.)

C. S. (Cecil Scott) Forester (1899-1966)

Forester departed from sea stories with "The Bedchamber Mystery" (*Cosmopolitan*, Oct. 1943; *Reader's Digest*, Feb. 1953) about three elderly spinsters sharing a house, one of whom shatters a china chamberpot under her weight and lacerates herself. The injured woman is embarrassed to call their doctor, Dr. Acheson, but they arrive on a plan and have the maid call him. Acheson arrives to find the victim in the middle of the floor and covered by an identity-concealing sheet with a hole in it to expose the injured region. The two other sisters are gone. Cooperating, he silently stitches up the wounds without asking questions or lifting up the sheet. Later, the sisters have Acheson over for dinner to thank him, and he notices that all three sisters have an extra cushion on their seats. Last line: "There was no knowing which of the sisters needed a cushion."

Evelyn Waugh (1903-1966)

Vile Bodies starts out by introducing several main characters as they get seasick on a rough English Channel crossing.

Samuel Beckett (1906-1989)

Waiting For Godot, Endgame, and others contain plenty of excremental puns, references, etc., but the standout is *Krapp's Last Tape,* about an old man who has fought a lifelong battle against constipation.

Jean Genet (1910-1986)

Genet's interest in bodily functions shows up in many of his works. *Our Lady of the Flowers* recounts a smell-oriented prisoner's limited world of farting, defecation, masturbation, and other solitary activi-

ties. Jean-Paul Sartre writes in his 1952 introduction, "No other book, not even *Ulysses,* brings us into such close physical contact with an author. Through the prisoner's nostrils we inhale his own odor." In *The Thief's Journal,* Genet discusses the unusual qualities of a compatriot's saliva and the pleasures of shitting in prison and mentions another thief's habit of "posting a watchman" (defecating) at the scenes of his crimes. Regarding his plays, Genet liked the idea of getting the bourgeoisie to pay high prices to come to the theater and be showered with scatological abuse. An example is *The Screens,* set during Algeria's war of independence (1954-1962), which features spitting, pissing, shitting, and a monologue about the equalizing effect of defecation.

Robertson Davies (1913-)

In *The Rebel Angels,* Professor Ozias Froats, known in the University community as the "Turd-Skinner," studies how people's shit might reflect their body type and temperament. His well-funded research involves regularly collecting feces from scores of subjects and examining slices of it under the microscope.

William S. Burroughs (1914-)

Along with drug addiction and hallucination, *Naked Lunch* makes frequent references to purulent discharges, excretion, coprophagy, pederasty, anal growths, unnecessary and messy surgical procedures, and ejaculation. As an "Atrophied Preface" placed toward the end of the disjointed novel explains, "*Naked Lunch* is a blueprint, a How-To Book . . . . Abstract concepts, bare as algebra, narrow down to a black turd or a pair of aging cajones."

Heinrich Boll (1917-1985)

In *Group Portrait With Lady,* Sister Rahel regularly inspects and keeps detailed records of the young schoolgirls' urine and feces, and uses these records to predict their scholastic achievement.

Gunter Grass (1927-)

The "Inspection of Feces" section of *The Flounder*

relates that the abbess Fat Gret inspects the feces of all novices and people seeking jobs in the kitchen. It also discusses the joys of communal shitting.

Hubert Selby Jr. (1928-)

Last Exit to Brooklyn describes in vivid detail a group of housewives sitting on a bench, picking boogers and scabs and farting while gossiping.

Milan Kundera (1929-)

In *The Unbearable Lightness of Being*, Kundera recalls that Stalin's son killed himself over refusing to reform his toilet habits while in a German POW camp during World War II, and then explains that kitsch, which exists in politics as well as in art, represents the denial of shit.

John (James) Osborne (1929-)

In *Luther*, Osborne accurately portrays Martin Luther as a foul-mouthed constipator, giving him lines such as, "I'm like a ripe stool in the world's straining anus, and at any moment we're about to let each other go."

Carlos Castaneda (1931-)

The Teachings of Don Juan: A Yaqui Way of Knowledge contains many hallucinogenically re-interpreted vomiting scenes. In one, for example, Carlos relates that during a peyote experience he felt, "unvoiced thoughts coming out of my mouth in a sort of liquid form. . .a pleasant flow of liquid words." He finds out later that he had thrown up about ten times, pissed uncontrollably, and gone into convulsions.

Sylvia Plath (1932-1963)

In *The Bell Jar*, the magazine staff all gets food poisoning and everyone starts throwing up. Betsy and Esther, interning there for the summer, barf together in their hotel room: "There is nothing like puking with somebody to make you old friends."

Philip Roth (1933-)

In *Portnoy's Complaint*, Alex Portnoy's girlfriend tells of a former lover who wanted to watch her defecate from underneath a glass tabletop (as Adolf Hitler and Nelson Rockefeller are said to have enjoyed). Meanwhile, Alex Portnoy discusses how no matter how fully he wipes himself, he still finds a wisp of feces stain on his jockey shorts. The novel also contains a famous discussion of teenage masturbation.

Amiri Baraka (LeRoi Jones) (1934-)

All of *The Toilet*, a harshly realistic play about teenage racial hostilities and the survival of the cruelest, takes place in a high school bathroom.

Thomas Pynchon (1937-)

In *Gravity's Rainbow*, Slothrop loses his harmonica down the toilet while throwing up and imagines following it down into the sewer system. Brigadier Pudding visits his mistress in the psychological warfare agency facility, and they go through their sex routine: she whips him, and then he drinks her urine, eats her feces, and masturbates.

Erica Jong (1942-)

In *Fear of Flying*, Isadora discusses how characteristics of different countries' toilets reflect national character.

Patrick Suskind (1949-)

The main character in *Perfume*, Grenouille, has an extremely acute sense of smell but no odor of his own. In his first attempt at creating a perfume to make him smell like a normal person, he begins with old cat shit.

Martin Amis (1949-)

In *Class*, Terry discusses how modern girls freely go to the lavatory, whereas in days gone by he used to imagine that ambulances took women to hospitals to defecate. Terry also describes the happenings in the nasty bathroom at work, with stalls so small that you're liable to accidently pull up the pants of the guy next to you instead of your own.

Seth Morgan (1949?-1990)

In *Homeboy*, Joe bleeds and collapses from pass-

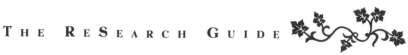

ing a "Yenshee baby," a boulder of impacted feces his recovering body tries to push out after years of constipating heroin addiction. Later, Kitty discovers Rings at a motel near Galveston, jumping out of a toilet-shaped cake for the Mid-South Plumbers Association convention.

Nicholson Baker (1957-)

In *The Mezzanine*, Howie reflects on his own piss-shyness in the office restroom and on workplace mensroom situations and protocols. In *Room Temperature*, Mike describes how, following their engagement, he and his wife began discussing their bowel movements with ever-increasing honesty and enthusiasm, how he experimented with target defecation as a boy, and how his revealing to his wife that he sometimes picks his nose in bed after she turns the light off could diminish her view of him and strain their relationship.

Bodily Functions in the Cinema

Nose Picking

The One And Only (1978)
Henry Winkler character, trying to be romantic, says to a potential date, "Do you pick your nose? I can't imagine a girl as pretty as you picking her nose." She looks up and replies, "I pick."

Traffic (France, 1972)
Artful montage of Mr. Hulot and other drivers picking their noses while stopped at intersections.

Revenge of the Nerds (1984)
"Booger" picks throughout film, doing it once to repulse opponent and win at arm wrestling.

Willie Wonka and the Chocolate Factory (1971)
Prissy little girl digs away while talking about what a nasty habit gum chewing is.

A King in New York (1973)
Charlie Chaplin character sees kid knead bread dough, stop to pick nose, and then continue kneading.

UHF (1989)
Stanley the janitor pulls out a big one while on TV.

Annie Hall (1977)
Kids in classroom during one of Alvy Singer's childhood flashbacks.

Das Boot (West Germany, 1982)
Demonstrating lack of privacy on U-boat, submariners dig away in full view.

Urine

National Lampoon's Animal House (1978)
Bluto absentmindedly relieves self on Pinto and Flounder's shoes.

Hair (1979)
Berger sees wedding announcement in newspaper he's peeing on, and the whole gang decides to attend.

National Lampoon's Vacation (1983)
Dog pees on sandwiches, but grandma eats one anyway.

Sweetie (New Zealand, 1990)
Sweetie pees out of open car door to avoid being left behind by her family's driving off.

Last Exit To Brooklyn (1990)
Father pees out window onto city sidewalk because daughter is using bathroom for a long time.

Reds (1982)
Alexander Berkman, in jail for shooting Henry Frick, has kidney disease. Another prisoner who sees him pee remarks, "He even pees red!"

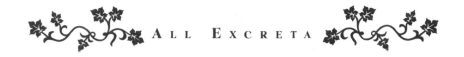

War Of The Roses (1989)
Oliver Rose pees on fish before it's brought to dinner table.

Richard Pryor Live In Concert (1978)
Pryor discusses how men and women differ when it comes to peeing in the woods.

The Natural History of Parking Lots (1990)
Older brother teaches protagonist L.A. folk rhyme, "I had the desire to pee on your tire. When I let it spill, it was fulfilled."

S.O.B. (1981)
Robert Webber character disrespectfully urinates in mortuary.

Caligula (1980)
Two women straddle and "golden shower" a dead man.

Europa, Europa (Germany/Poland/France, 1991)
In the penultimate scene, Solomon and Isaac urinate together out in the open after Solomon "goes public" with his Jewish identity.

Major League (1989)
Manager pees on Dorn's contract when he claims exemption from exercises.

Prospero's Books (Britain, 1991)
Ariel's young boy persona urinates continuously through most of the opening sequence.

Vomit

Monty Python's The Meaning Of Life (Britain, 1983)
Famous "Mr. Creosote" sketch depicting voluminous regurgitation by enormous man after enormous meal. Seen by pop culture eggheads as early example of antagonistic, "post-funny" comedy, a la Andy Kaufman.

Harold and Maude (1971)

Harold barfs and then kisses Shelley Duvall character.

This Is Spinal Tap (1984)
Band members discuss the origin of the vomit an ex-drummer choked to death on.

Stand By Me (1986)
Wil Wheaton character tells exaggerated pie-eating contest turned "barf-o-rama" story.

Dead-Bang (1989)
Don Johnson character throws up all over bad guy and threatens to puke on him again if he refuses to talk.

Wild At Heart (1990)
Lula's mother smears face with lipstick and vomits in rage.

The Witches of Eastwick (1987)
Several cherry-puking scenes.

Erik the Viking (Britain, 1989)
Seasickness rampant just before meeting "Sun" monster.

Life Is Sweet (Britain, 1991)
Bulimic binge-purge episode by troubled daughter in her bedroom.

Farts

Airplane! (1980)
The pilot is affected by mild food poisoning.

Murder By Death (1976)
Scene with Agatha Christie type character and her servant: "Do you smell gas?" "I can't help it; I'm old."

Blazing Saddles (1974)
Bean-eating cowboys toot up a storm by the old campfire.

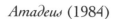 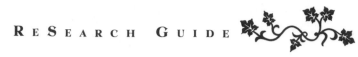
Amadeus (1984)
Mozart rips one mockingly after caricaturing Salieri at the piano.

Amarcord (Italy, 1974)
Fellini-as-a-young-man's grandfather relaxes fully after dinner.

The Hollywood Knights (1980)
Newbomb Turk farts while singing "Volare."

The Canterbury Tales (Italy, 1972)
Pasolini commits Chaucer's "The Miller's Tale" to film.

Le Grande Bouffe (Italy/France, 1973)
Michel Piccoli character farts himself to death.

Fanny and Alexander (Sweden, 1982)
Uncle Karlchen astonishes children by blowing out candles.

Polyester (1981)
With "Smell-O-Rama" technology (a card with scratch 'n' sniffs numbered to match numbers flashed on screen), director John Waters gives moviegoers a more complete illusion of a fart.

9 ½ Weeks (1986)
Mickey Rourke character pays $1 to hear a kid fart the *Jaws* theme.

Madonna: Truth Or Dare (1991)
Madonna recites the following poem:
A fart is a chemical substance,
It comes from a place called "bum,"
It penetrates through trousers
And lands with a risible hum.
To fart, to fart, 'tis no disgrace,
For it gives the body ease,
It warms the blankets on cold winter nights
And suffocates all the fleas.

Feces

Mad Magazine's Up the Academy (1980)
Turd in punch bowl.

Where's Poppa? (1970)
A young nurse describes how on her wedding night, her husband defecated while they made love. She asked, "How could you?" and he replied, "Doesn't everyone?"

Dances With Wolves (1990)
Union soldiers wipe selves with pages torn from the Kevin Costner character's journal.

The Magic Christian (Britain, 1970)
Final scene shows people diving for cash in vat of animal excrement and entrails.

Twilight of the Cockroaches (Japan, 1989)
"Talking Turd" character.

City Lights (1931)
Charlie Chaplin character, working as a street sweeper, sees parade of horses go down street, followed by an elephant.

Monty Python and the Holy Grail (Britain, 1975)
Frenchmen in castle empty chamberpots on heads of King Arthur and his men.

Jabberwocky (Britain, 1977)
Massive Jabberwock dump found in woods.

Three Men and a Cradle (France, 1986)
Recurrent theme of diapers needing changing.

The Last Emperor (1987)
Court doctor closely examines Child-Emperor's stools.

Padre, Padrone (Italy, 1977)
Goat keeps crapping in milk pail while being milked.

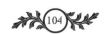

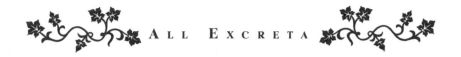

Weird Science (1985)
Older brother turned into pile of shit.

The Holy Mountain (Germany, 1974)
Alchemist converts feces into gold.

Kiss Of The Spider Woman (1985)
In prison, Raul Julia character has the runs from being poisoned by William Hurt character.

Raw (1987)
Eddie Murphy discusses his stools.

Harper Valley P.T.A. (1978)
Truckload of manure dumped into convertible.

Back To The Future (1985)
Truckload of manure dumped into convertible.

Back To The Future II (1989)
Truckload of manure dumped into convertible.

Toilets

2001: A Space Odyssey (1968)
In what director Kubrick said was the film's only intentional joke, Dave reads instructions for Zero Gravity toilet.

True Love (1989)
During wedding reception, bride cries in toilet stall after argument with groom.

Witness (1985)
Amish boy witnesses murder in men's room.

The Bad News Bears in Breaking Training (1977)
Hefty kid sits on can eating from bucket of fried chicken.

Porky's II: The Next Day (Canada, 1983)
Tommy sends snake thru the toilet to scare Miss Ballbricker.

Robocop (1987)
Confrontation in john between Corporation V.P. and young upstart; scared exec onlooker forgets to zip up and wets self.

Lethal Weapon II (1989)
Danny Glover character sits on booby-trapped toilet.

Letter to Brezhnev (Britain, 1986)
Two main characters talk and change into party clothes in stall.

Prick Up Your Ears (1987)
Joe Orton and total strangers have sex in the dark in a public men's room.

The Discreet Charm of the Bourgeoisie (France, 1972)
Guests sit on toilets at "dinner" table, chatting and defecating. They pass toilet paper to one another on silver trays. From time to time, guests excuse themselves and go into a small room to quickly eat something.

Assassination (1987)
Woman opens door on Bronson character reading newspaper on airplane toilet.

Husbands (1970)
John Cassavetes, Peter Falk, and Ben Gazzara characters drunkenly male-bond in men's room, urinating, defecating, and vomiting all the while.

Fame (1980)
Boys in boys' room spy through hole into girls' room; stalls collapse, exposing unconcerned music student practicing french horn on toilet.

Fun With Dick and Jane (1977)
Jane Fonda character wipes self.

Something Wild (1986)
Melanie Griffith character wipes self.

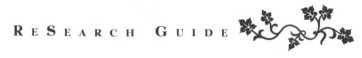

Everything

(Note that most of these are either High Art or Low Comedy)

Caddyshack (1980)

Suspected turd in swimming pool turns out to be candy bar; guys in bushes take bets over whether little Spalding would pick his nose, and then if he would eat it; Al farts in Bushwood dining room; Ty takes a leak on the golf course; little Spalding pukes in the doctor's Porsche.

Pink Flamingos (1974)

Wrapped turd given as gift, man at party shows off uniquely expressive anus, Divine eats freshly dropped poodle poop (one continuous shot, no special effects) and almost barfs.

Shakes the Clown (1992)

In opening scene, Shakes gets peed on and then barfs. He throws up on a number of other occasions as well.

Salt, Saliva, Sperm and Sweat (Australia, 1988)

Four days of a man's life as told through his bodily fluids. Lots of close-ups. Glass toilet bowl.

The Cook, the Thief, His Wife, and Her Lover (Britain, 1990)

Albert Spica and his gang smear man with dog excrement and force him to eat some; then Albert urinates on him; later, one of Albert's goons pukes at the dinner table. Albert's wife and a gynecologist begin an affair in a ladies' room, and Albert kicks open stalls looking for them

The Exorcist (1973)

Linda Blair character barfs, urinates on carpet, etc.

History of the World Part I (1981)

Emperor Nero farts while sitting on his throne; critic pees on cave painting.

Caveman (1981)

Neanderthal runs away from newly-discovered fire, his farts igniting and shooting flame; name sought for massive Tyrannosaurus turd; Barbara Bach character thrown in pile.

Sweet Movie (Yugoslavia, 1974)

Much scatological material in extreme close-up.

Meet the Feebles (New Zealand)

In one scene, Louie the Fly eats feces out of Harry the Hare's toilet and remarks "Oh—carrots! It must be one of yours, Harry."

Bad Taste (New Zealand)
Gross Out (1991)

Two movies intentionally made to be as disgusting as possible.

Dr. Strangelove (1964)

Col. Jack D. Ripper (Sterling Hayden) feels that fluoridation is a Communist plot to destroy our precious bodily fluids. To maintain his "Purity Of Essence" (which he equates with "Peace On Earth"), he only drinks branch water and grain alcohol, and he denies his "essence" to any woman he consorts with.

Numerous Historical Applications of Excrement

As most people know, farmers have used animal and human excrement for fertilizer since agriculture began. Many also are aware that dung has been used as plaster and mortar, and as a fuel for cooking and heating. But these are just a few of the many uses people throughout history and around the world have found for excrement, in areas as diverse as agriculture, cloth-making, and cosmetics.

Farmers everywhere have traditionally fertilized crops with dung, but in some countries, new hybrid seeds which grow only in oil-based fertil-

izer are replacing the manure-growing ones cultivated for millennia. The chemical fertilizer industry has encouraged this potentially hazardous switch, and for this reason, Reginald Reynolds calls this industry "one of the biggest rackets in the world." Meanwhile, Dan Sabbath reports that Russia has had the good sense to establish a bank of so-called "archaic" seeds for the day when petroleum supplies are exhausted.

Farmers use manure in other ways as well. They incubate eggs in it, burn it as a smudge to protect their crops from insects and frost, and smear it on the teats of dams to hasten weaning.

Tanners use both dung and urine to prepare hides. Dyers use urine to bleach and dye cloth or to fix the colors of woolen fabrics. Some traditional European recipes produce blue, violet, and bluish-red dyes from stale urine and lichens. Pliny notes that urine is also good for removing ink stains.

Urine and feces were also used to prepare smoking materials. In many areas, animal dung itself is a traditional smoke. Human feces was used to cure tobacco in the U.S., and the traditional cigar manufacturing process in Cuba included soaking the tobacco leaves in the urine of young girls. Meanwhile, in China, hen dung was used to cut opium.

Urine was probably the first soap, and has been used everywhere as a cleaning product. The oxidation of urine produces ammonia compounds, which are standard agents for dissolving fats. The English word "chamber lye" specifically refers to stale urine when used as a cleanser. Urine, dung, and dung ashes have been used to wash dishes. In addition, urine has been used to launder clothes, shampoo and condition hair, and soften hands. Jonathan Swift notes women's use of puppy urine as a general-purpose beauty lotion.

Ancient Romans bleached their hair with pigeon dung, and used dung and dung ashes as a hair dressing. Dung is also a common ingredient in folk cures for baldness and dandruff. The Romans used urine as a mouthwash and dentifrice, as noted by Catullus. In China, the preferred mouthwash was baby urine.

Human and animal urine has been employed in the manufacture of salt, phosphorus, saltpeter, and sal ammoniac. Galen describes a recipe for jeweler's cement that contains the urine of a child. Privy fumes have been used to restore the color of coral and the odor of musk. Urine mixed with carbon dust has been used as a tattoo pigment. Eskimos created steam baths by urinating on hot stones in an enclosed tent.

Second Kings 6:25, which reports that during a great famine and siege of Samaria, one quarter kab (about a pint) of dove's dung cost five pieces of silver. Some authors have pointed to this reference as evidence that the Samarians found dove's dung useful. Scholars explain, however, that "dove's dung" is an old Arab term for dried garbanzo beans.

Excrement in Food and Drink

Food becomes excrement, and in this way the two are closely related, but in many old recipes, excrement also becomes food. Many foods we like also remind us of excrement, and we sometimes even name them or present them in ways that reinforce the connection.

In his *Concept of Repression* (1921), the inventive but marginal Indian psychologist Girindrashekhar Bose argues that many of our foods smell like our excretions. Certain cheeses, onions, and the durian fruit of Southeast Asia smell like feces; cucumber smells like semen; asafetida, a resin used in condiments and chutnies, smells like farts; and vinegar smells like sweat. He also asserts that tobacco smells like decomposing urine; and that cabbage, salted hilsa fish (a Bengali delicacy) and roasted meat smell like decomposing bodies.

Bose may be stretching things a bit, but undeniably some foods, often those considered delicacies, do resemble body products. Novelist Witold Gombrowicz writes in his diary that breakfast at the Hermitage in France smelled of, "forgive me, a very luxurious water closet." It's hard to imag-

ine a more elegant meal than one consisting entirely of the products of fungal growth, fermentation, and decay-all processes associated with excrement: well-aged beef, mushrooms, truffles, cheeses, and wine, especially a late-harvest vintage. And as Salvador Dali once told an interviewer, "There is nothing gastronomically more eye-appealing than the shade of loose stools."

Sausages in particular have a strong association with feces, due to their shape and because they're made by stuffing intestines. We've already noted that in Europe, some quasi-religious ceremonies use sausages to symbolize turds. Along the same lines, the wife of the Elector of Hanover wrote in 1694 to Liselotte, her niece, "If meat makes shit, it is also true that shit makes meat . . . . Isn't it so that on the most delicate tables shit is served in stews. . .the black puddings, the chitterlings, the sausages, are they not stews in shit sacks?"

A number of foods less directly related to excrement have scatological names. "Pumpernickel" comes from old German words for farting (pumpern) and the devil (nickel), the implication being that the bread is so tough to digest, it would make a devil fart, or it makes you fart like the devil (scholars question the story that Napoleon first called the bread an apple for his horse, a "pomme pour Nicole"). The Germans also bake rosewater shortbread biscuits called "Nonnenfürzchen" (nun's farts) and (as previously mentioned) make little candies in the shape of a man squatting and defecating a large coin. Freud had a field day with this candy figurine, called the "Ducatenscheisser."

Recently, the food-excrement connection was reasserted by The Klo ("The Toilet"), a popular Berlin pub that used toilets as chairs, offered toilet paper as napkins, and served hot entrees such as "sausage and cabbage in a chamber pot" to accompany the beer.

But going beyond mere references and resemblances, excrement itself has been used as food all over the world. We've discussed urine-drinking in religious ceremonies and upon social occasions. Hindus traditionally drink cow urine for good luck. Central Africans mix cow urine in with their milk. Chinooks prepared "Chinook Olives" by soaking acorns in urine for five months. Before yeast was introduced, European bakers may have used urine in breadmaking. The O.E.D.'s entry for "chamber lye" asserts that taverns extended cheap ale with urine. Cheesemakers in Germany and Switzerland used urine in their cheese. According to a 1888 letter to John G. Bourke, a storekeeper in Berlin was punished for using the urine of young girls to make his cheese richer and more piquant, but people continued buying and enjoying it anyway.

North American natives made a broth from rabbit and caribou dung. Near Lake Superior, they boiled rabbit feces with their wild rice. Australian aborigines prepared a sweet beverage from the excrement of the green beetle. Persians smoked melons with pigeon dung. In Siberia, Central Africa, and North America, cooks prepared intestines without emptying them first. Often, however, the cooked intestine contents themselves would not be eaten.

Some fetishists, insane people, and children (particularly children who have soiled their beds and expect punishment) have eaten human feces straight. Bourke cites two cases of children who had done this and then been asked what it tasted like. Both answered that it had a stinking and somewhat sweet taste.

Bourke also cites an 1886 article from the *General Homeopathic Journal* about a Parisian bakery that unwittingly used raw sewage:

The neighbors of an establishment famous for its excellent bread and pastries complained again and again of the disgusting smells which prevailed therein and which penetrated into their dwellings. The appearance of cholera finally lent force to these complaints, and the sanitary inspectors who were sent to investigate the matter found there was a connection between the water closets of these dwellings and the reservoir supplying the bakery. This connection was cut off at once, but the immediate result thereof was a perceptible deterioration of the quality of the bread. Chemists have evidently no difficulty in demonstrating that water impregnated with "extract of water closet" has the peculiar property of causing dough to rise particularly high, thereby imparting the pleasing appearance and flavor which characterize sumptuous bread.

In another set of practices which anthropologists term the "Second Harvest," people sift through their own feces or the feces of animals and pick out for consumption grains or seeds which have passed through undigested. Lower Californians would eat the seeds of the pitahaya cactus, collect them from their stools, and then roast, grind, and re-ingest them. Hindu Brahmins considered whole grains found in cow dung to be sacred.

A European custom had young women prepare "cockle-bread," a food intended to excite men's passion, by sitting on dough and wiggling around to knead it, sometimes reciting a rhyme in the process ("Up with my heels and down with my head/And this is the way to mould cockle-bread" is an example). One scholar, Edward Lucie-Smith, has written that cockle-bread was made with menstrual blood.

Sanitation and Excrement Through Western History

Rural life presents few sanitation problems. On lands wandered by nomads or cultivated by traditional farmers, life forms of the food-chain balance each other so that disposal of animal wastes is not a concern. In fact, these wastes help the plants grow. On the other hand, large metropolitan areas with millions of inhabitants, no farmland, and "Please Keep Off The Grass" parks have a lot of shit to deal with. Sanitation is an urban problem.

So it's not surprising that the first advances in sanitation and plumbing came with the first cities, which grew in the "cradles of civilization" such as the Nile valley, home of the Egyptians, the Tigris and Euphrates river valleys a thousand miles east in present-day Iraq, home of the Sumerians, Akkadians, and Mesopotamians, and the Indus river valley a thousand miles east in present-day Pakistan, home of the Indus civilization.

These cities began to spring up between 5000 and 3000 B.C., during the Copper Age (Chalcolithic Era), the relatively short period between the Neolithic Era when people hadn't yet started working in metal, and the Bronze Age, when word had gotten around that adding tin or arsenic to the copper makes a better product.

Excavations of Mohenjo-Daro, one of the main Indus cities, have uncovered chutes and flues from high floors emptying into bins in the street dating from around 3000 B.C. Privies from the same era have been unearthed at Tell Asman, in the ancient Sumerian city of Ashnunnak. Later, when Sargon the Great had conquered and united the entire Tigris-Euphrates region, around 2300 B.C., he built himself a huge palace with six Western-style (high seat) toilets. Later still, the ancient Egyptians had drains of hammered copper. Around 2000 B.C. the royal palace at Knossos, capital of the Minoan civilization on Crete, had a marble latrine with a removable plug and a cistern of water above for flushing. Knossos also had a complex sewer system.

A great advance of scale happened much later under the Tarquins, three visionary kings of the pre-empire city of Rome who ruled during the sixth century B.C. and united the city with public works including the Cloaca Maxima, an enormous open sewer fourteen feet wide and seventeen-and-a-half feet high. In another major project nearly 200 years later, the sewer was covered.

Early Rome and the Roman Empire dealt with body products in the political as well as technological spheres. In 282 B.C. an angry mob in Tarentum, a prosperous Greek city in southern Italy that resisted Rome's encroaching influence, pelted the Roman ambassador Posthumus with dung. The ambassador responded that it would take a lot of Tarentine blood to wash the stains from his toga. War started, and Rome defeated

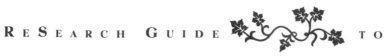

Tarentum and made it a province.

Centuries later, in a scene reminiscent of *Monty Python's Life Of Brian*, a Roman soldier in Jerusalem farted toward some Jews celebrating Passover. The insult immediately resulted in a riot that killed 10,000 people and was one of the events leading up to the First Jewish War in A.D. 67-68.

At home, Vespasian, who ruled from 69 to 79, improved Rome with polished marble public urinals. The government sold the contents of these urinals to dyers and fullers who bleached cloth with it, making the amenities a source of revenue as well as comfort (interestingly, the Romans wrote obscene poetry on the walls of their public toilets just as we do today). Meanwhile, copper receptacles called "gastra" were installed along the rural roads for the convenience of travelers, and the contents of these went to local agriculture. China had the same system.

Each Roman public toilet had a bucket full of salt water with a sponge on a stick in it for wiping. As mentioned previously, Seneca's Epistle No 70 describes the suicide of a German slave who rammed one of these sticks down his own throat.

As Rome declined, fell, and gave way to the Catholic Church as the major power in Europe, three people exemplary of this shift all met similar scatological fates. In 222, Emperor Heliogabalus was assassinated in a latrine—he had ruled Rome for four years and was known for entertaining dinner guests by burning slaves to death inside an enormous metal statue of a bull. In 336, the Greek theologian Arius, author of the now-heretical, non-Trinitarian doctrine that Jesus Christ and God the Father were separate entities, was also murdered in the toilet. James Joyce refers to this event in *Ulysses*. Finally, in 461, after the Roman Empire had fallen, Pope Leo the Great (known as "Saint Leo") was also killed at toilet. Leo had been a major opponent of Arian Christianity, which was the Catholic Church's main political threat during his papacy.

Of the Middle Ages, Lawrence Wright notes, "For a thousand years Europe went unwashed." Indeed, from 395 when Rome fell, ending an era in which people socialized at public baths and

cooperated in keeping the cities clean and orderly, until the mid-18th Century, the beginning of what Alain Corbin calls the "olfactory revolution," Europeans bathed very little.

The new era in history brought toilet-related politics of its own. In Tewkesbury, Gloucester, England in 1259, a Jew fell into a cesspit on a Saturday and asked in observance of the Sabbath not to be helped out until the next day. The Earl of Gloucester heard this and commanded that he not be fished out on Sunday either so that he would observe the Christian Sabbath as well with similar reverence. On Monday they discovered him dead.

In 1596, Sir John Harington, a member of the Elizabethan court illegitimately descended from King Henry VIII, wrote *The Metamorphosis of Ajax, A New Discourse on a Stale Subject*. The title makes a pun on "Ajax" a Greek hero in the *Iliad*, and "A jakes," meaning a toilet. It also plays with the two meanings of "stale:" not fresh, and the urine of livestock. Harington's Rabelais-influenced celebration of the scatological not only inspired imitations such as the anonymous *Ulysses Upon Ajax* of a few years later, but more astonishingly, contained a complete plan for the first valve toilet. A few were built in royal palaces, but because water back then was hand-carried in, not piped, the thirsty little invention didn't attain widespread use until 200 years later.

Throughout the smelly millennium, Europeans made a few new additions to excretory product-disposal methods. Cesspools gained popularity, often as the endpoint of sewer systems far from convenient rivers or gorges, and cesspool-clearers often dumped the sewage into gutters to save trips to the dump. Castles had privies hanging out over moats or pits below, explaining the long tapered stains we see trailing down from small protruding rooms on castle walls today. Some monasteries built on the ocean had sea-level privies flushed twice daily by the tides. In Madrid, Edinburgh, and other cities, men would walk or ride carts through the streets renting out the use of a portable privy, or simply a bucket and a shielding cloak, announcing their presence to the public by calling "Wha wants me for a bewbee?" (an Edinburgh cry) or the local language equivalent. But one of the most popular ways of disposing of night soil in Europe's cities was simply to dump it into the street, where it would mix with the horse droppings and whatever else was there. This practice generated another bit of colorful Edinburgh slang which remains as one of our language's wackiest and best-loved words: gardyloo. Residents corrupted the French "Gardez l'eau" (beware the water) into this warning call they politely yelled before emptying chamberpots into the street from upper windows; Hogarth depicted the process in his "Night" etching, from *Four Times of the Day*. Any pedestrians passing beneath would respond with "Haud yer han" (hold your hand) to delay the shower and then hurry away.

Excrement was all over the cities of Europe, in its streets, its rivers, streams, ditches, cesspools, and even in its buildings. But another factor contributing to the special atmosphere Europe had during this time was infrequent bathing. Both scientific and religious thought discouraged personal cleanliness. Doctors condemned excess water use and connected strong smells with "animality" and hence vigor and health. Many held onto the ancient belief that excrement and strong odors healed (partially true; hydrogen sulfide (H_2S), the pungent "rotten egg" gas sewage can produce, is a disinfectant). Many doctors recommended standing over a privy and breathing deeply first thing in the morning! Authorities even tried to combat London's plague of 1664 with the power of stench by ordering all cesspools opened. Throughout Europe's many devastating plagues, the suffering populations viewed water and bathing more often as a culprit rather than a solution.

Meanwhile, the early church condemned bathing as a time-wasting luxury and regarded the public baths, most of them left over from the intemperate Romans, as hotbeds of sin. Benedict, the sixth century saint who founded the Benedictine monastic order, wrote, "to those that are well, and especially to the young, bathing shall seldom be permitted." Following this sort of ad-

vice, the Master at one of the colleges at Cambridge vetoed construction of student baths, reasoning that the young men would only be around for eight weeks at a time. Moreover, it was felt, dirt contributed to the beauty of peasant women's complexions by blocking out the sun. People also believed that the dirtier children were, the healthier they were. Body odor expressed people's individuality, their national character, trade, dietary preferences, and other traits, and as anyone who has ever read a t-shirt or a bumper sticker knows, individual expression to the world at large is important in our culture. Up to a point, Europeans actually liked stinks and filth; they were comforting and familiar—a part of the people. All the same, heat and other unfavorable conditions must have occasionally made odors difficult for even the most filth-loving butcher, tanner, or cesspool clearer to bear. Perhaps the rapid spread of tobacco-smoking in Europe might be partially due to its ability to mask odors and dull the sense of smell.

By many accounts, when Europeans began colonizing the rest of the world, the indigenous populations were taken aback by how bad they smelled. Of course, some of these first impressions must have been of Europeans coming right off ships, the stinkiest places of all due to the lack of fresh water, but Europe's big cities were awful too, especially their prisons and hospitals. Prison ventilation was poor, there were no bathing facilities, and prisoners had to "go to the bathroom" on the floors of their cells. The scene in Beethoven's *Fidelio* in which the prisoners, let up out of their dungeon, break into song about how wonderful the sunlight and fresh air are, dramatizes this aspect of prison life. In his *The State of the Prisons* (1784), John Howard writes that on the somber occasion when the Comte de Struensee was taken out of a dungeon to be beheaded, his words were, "Oh, the happiness of breathing fresh air!"

Hospitals stank from excrement, decaying corpses, excised tissues, gangrenous limbs, infectious discharges, and the like. As with prisons, the stench permeated the walls-the buildings

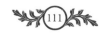

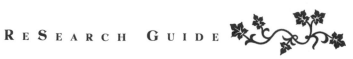

themselves oozed a reeking miasma.

The many prisons, hospitals, cesspools, butcher shops, tanneries, fulleries, polluted waterways, and the sheer density of population made strong smells inescapable in major cities such as Paris. In his 1788 portrait of the City of Light, Louis Sébastien Mercier notes that while it may be the center of science, arts, fashion, and taste, Paris also stands as the center of stench.

To its credit, the pervasiveness of odor had an equalizing effect on the population, as Maugham discusses in *On a Chinese Screen*. Rich and poor alike lived unwashed lives, surrounded by odor. Even the palace at Versailles stank, and it was out in the countryside. Servants and guests pissed and shat in its courtyards and gardens and even in the hallways, empty rooms, and corners of the palace building itself. Excrement that did make it into the sewer system often ended up in a cesspool next door. In the city of Versailles, women even urinated during church services; Louis Bourdaloue, a Jesuit preacher active there during the 17th Century, delivered sermons so long that they inspired the invention of the "bourdaloue," a lipless, oblong porcelain vessel women congregants would secrete (and secrete into) beneath their skirts.

The latter half of the 18th Century brought not only national and industrial revolution but olfactory and sanitary revolution as well. Before this time, although common wisdom instructed people to specifically avoid the "smell of death" during plagues, strong odors from various places around town were simply considered a part of the landscape. By our standards, city dwellers lived in a world of intolerable stench, but at the time, it wasn't perceived as a problem. Meanwhile, scientists who were investigating the airborne transmission of infection did so in purely abstract terms, with few references to the sense of smell.

Around 1760, however, these researchers began associating characteristic smells with the infections, contaminations, fermentations, putrefactions, and other biological processes they observed, and the nose soon became an important tool for the study of these processes. Doctors and chemists began experimenting with odors, focusing largely on notions of good and bad air and mysterious vapors (germs hadn't yet been linked to disease). They collected farts, gases from bathwater and corpses, and other types of "airs" to discover the effects of inhaling them, and found that putrid air carries infection and, almost equally significantly, affects one's own personal odor—a threatening prospect during an age that embraced individuality as a new ideal. These newly-perceived threats caused urban populations to shift interpretations and to perceive strong odors, particularly fecal odors, as life-threatening and hence intolerable.

Soon neighborhood residents began fighting not-in-my-backyard battles against slaughterhouses, tanneries, prisons, hospitals, cesspools, and cemeteries. People gave speeches, argued, and filed lawsuits in an attempt to clear their neighborhood air. The stronger, more public works-oriented governments that had come into being responded to these new anti-odor sentiments and engineered the sanitary revolution.

Hospitals started changing sheets and clothes, prisons replaced doors with grilles, cities maintained cesspools more diligently, paved streets, installed drains, and rebuilt sewer systems; the new consciousness put a lot of people to work. Fans were invented and soon became popular. Another deodorization tactic people used was fumigation, which usually meant pouring vinegar over a hot shovel. They didn't know this at the time, but as the vinegar cloud deodorized, it also killed the germs it contacted. Back in the 1670's, van Leeuwenhoek had discovered under the microscope that vinegar kills microbes, but he never associated them with either odor or disease.

Deodorization immediately took on a political/social significance. Its strongest supporters came from the new middle class (the poor distrusted and rejected these goody-goody nouveau-riche upstarts meddling with their lives, placing more trust in the aristocracy which was initially fairly indifferent). With deodorization, the bourgeoisie effectively made odor a new way of distinguishing and distancing themselves from the poor.

Some poor people, meanwhile, simply disagreed with the aims of the movement, finding stale air cozy and reassuring. Other more combative proletarians openly embraced their new distinguishing feature, reveling in its ability to spook the bourgeoisie, thumbing their noses at this uptight new class by revitalizing traditionally scatological public rites such as the Shrovetide carnival and the Feast of Fools, and by peppering their speech with vulgar words high-minded elements in society had been trying to abolish from the language for decades.

Predictably, a rebellious segment of the intellectual elite co-opted the masses' vulgar anti-bourgeois stance. Gustave Flaubert championed this posture as a young man. He and his friends always ended their letters to each other with mock-polite scatological valedictions. In one letter written in his early twenties, Flaubert urged a companion to challenge conventional manners: "Let diarrhea drip into your boots, piss from the window, shout out 'shit,' defecate in full view, fart hard, blow your cigar smoke in people's faces...belch in people's faces."

Schools began teaching deodorization techniques, and poor people whose only previous exposure to deodorized environments had been in hospitals, prisons, and barracks began adopting the measures themselves. In 1823, someone discovered that lime chloride in water was antiseptic, and it soon became indispensable.

Resistance died hard, however. Rumors flew that the use of chlorine was a mass homicide plot against the poor by the elite. In 1832, Parisian ragpickers demonstrated against municipal sanitary measures by rioting and burning dungcarts. A few doctors continued to champion the therapeutic value of feces, despite the new understanding of infection. It was a losing battle, however. Following public sentiment, public hygiene standards were established, and engineers and city governments began designing and building an infrastructure and sewage systems to uphold them.

The final blow was perhaps struck in 1881 when Louis Pasteur saved livestock from anthrax through inoculation, demonstrating the germ theory in a way everyone could understand. This boosted public support for sanitary reform considerably, eliminating nearly all remaining opposition.

Much great building occurred during the nineteenth century, changing the urban atmosphere so completely that young residents of the better-served areas associated smells with the countryside, not the city—a clear testament to the engineers' Herculean achievement. The technical challenges were divided into two areas: big-thinking civil engineers worked on vast municipal water and sewage networks, while tinkerer and inventor types developed bathroom fixtures, the most complicated and interesting being the flush toilet.

The big question on the sewer system side had to do with basic approach. Two different strategies evolved: closed-circuit and torrent. Closed-circuit systems completely seal sewage off from any environmental contact until it reaches the treatment plant or the ocean. In these systems, sewage remains in sealed pipes for long periods of time, putrefying and breeding anaerobic bacteria (as found inside a botulism-infected can). Any leaks or repair work releases dangerous amounts of the poisonous toxin.

Torrent systems, on the other hand, keep the sewage moving to avoid putrefaction until it dilutes into a stream or river or reaches filter beds in the ground. Leakage is less of a problem, because keeping the sewage moving and limiting its time in the pipe prevents germs from multiplying. Some smaller cities in Belgium and France installed closed-circuit systems, but engineers felt that larger versions of these systems would be unworkable. Big cities in Germany, England, Poland, and the U.S. installed torrent systems successfully, and they have been the model ever since.

Meanwhile, the toilet, being something tinkerable-with (unlike a large municipal sewer system), developed through incremental improvements rather than debate and projection. Many steps in its evolution came before the world was ready for them, but by the late 19th century, water and sewage systems were widely installed and ready to go. Harington had invented the toilet in

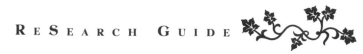

1596. In the 1770's, Alexander Cummings and Joseph Bramah improved it with a gooseneck trap, and slider or crank flush mechanisms, but not until the ascendancy of Thomas Crapper during the Victorian Era were large percentages of the population willing (and financially flush enough) to install modern toilets in their homes.

The Victorians redesigned plumbing in a grand style, equipping buildings with a spectrum of variously shaped and ornamented toilets far exceeding even the range available today. Toilet installation proliferated in American cities and towns as well, especially after Henry Wadsworth Longfellow installed one in his house in 1840. But the U.S.'s sparser, more rural population retained the outdoor privy as its primary elimination venue, long after Western Europe's cities had gone all-toilet.

In 1889 the Eiffel Tower opened, marking the completion over a century of unprecedented building in Europe. Providing adequate bathroom water pressure at the top of the then-World's Tallest Building was an engineering feat in itself. The first to officially use the bathroom was King Edward VII, who tested it at the tower's inauguration. Many who followed him were disappointed, however, by the frosted glass windows which made impossible a uniquely pleasurable aerial view.

Intermittently, the West enjoyed several boom times during the following forty years. This prosperity had the usual effect of inspiring people to create luxury—even entertainment—out of necessity, in the bathroom as well as the dining and bed rooms. New, more open attitudes and a fun-loving, faddish generation of young people also helped make the 1920's a boom time for bathroom novelties and toilet humor. Jokes in the jakes were nothing new; during the American Revolution, for example, some English water closets featured portraits of George Washington, fear being a known inducement to defecation. Later, novelty English chamberpots were manufactured with portraits of Napoleon in the bottoms. But the Twenties brought a flurry of toilet gadgets. Some devices would trigger chimes, confetti showers, or music when the "victim" unrolled some toilet paper. Reynolds tells of a gentleman who rigged a toilet seat to play the National Anthem as soon as anyone sat down, compelling the unfortunate to immediately stand back up. Probably the most elaborate toilet gag of the era was staged by a Hollywood producer who built a backyard privy whose walls fell down when the guest flushed!

The Great Depression brought cutbacks on bathroom extravagances. The men's room in New York's Grand Central Station had three toilet sections: five-cent and ten-cent pay toilet sections, and the free toilets. During the Thirties, the yearly income from the pay sections stayed at one-half of its 1929 level. Nevertheless, the free toilet section did offer a small extravagance that retained its popularity: a coin-operated peep show machine featuring Sally Rand, the era's most popular stripper.

Cutbacks on bathroom extravagances didn't mean cutbacks on bathrooms, however. Widespread poverty and a large homeless population demanded more public rest facilities then ever before. In 1934 alone, super-developer Robert Moses opened up 145 public toilets in New York City. In 1940, the city's Mayor Fiorello LaGuardia ordered weekly inspections of the 1,676 working subway station toilets, and according to the final report, all but a few were clean. Those were the days.

In the early days of commercial aviation after World War II, some lucky passengers were able to enjoy a pleasure denied Eiffel tower visitors. For transatlantic flights, the tail turrets originally built for gunners on Liberator aircraft were converted into toilets, and according to firsthand accounts, the panoramic views from these airborne privies remain unmatched, even today. Another spectacular airborne toilet was launched entirely by accident in a Palestinian encampment in 1947. Someone tried to rid a latrine of rats by pouring paraffin laced with DDT into the pit, and lighting it with a match. The explosive combination of paraffin, sewer gases, and fire blew the facility sky-high. Incredibly, no one was seriously hurt, not even the perpetrator, but fragments of toilet paper were drifting down from the sky for four hours afterwards!

Much effort was put into silencing the toilets of Westminster Abbey before the coronation of Queen Elizabeth II in 1952. The Royal Guard and BBC audio technicians equipped with decibel meters ensured that even all the church's toilets flushing at once would not be heard during the moment of silence when the queen's head would receive the crown.

In 1963, Brazilian longshoreman struck for an extra 20% "shame pay" for handling cargo such as water closets and sanitary supplies.

The CIA has tapped plumbing used by foreign dignitaries and others, Brezhnev and King Farouk being two examples, and run chemical tests on the contents, searching for the presence of anything suspicious or otherwise informative. The operation requires one agent stationed inside the restroom to signal which facility the dignitary uses.

A Japanese toilet was developed in 1989 to conduct these sorts of tests automatically, and not just on dignitaries. Toto Ltd., Omran Corporation, and Nippon Telegraph and Telephone collaborated to create an "intelligent toilet" that analyzes urine, displaying on a screen concentrations of sugar, protein, and urobilinogen. It can also test and display heart rate and blood pressure with the help of a sensor unit that takes the occupant's left index finger. The toilet can store the examination results in memory or send them to a printer, and NTT officials foresee hooking up systems to a communications network to enable them to send reports directly to clinics and hospitals, pushing the Information Age's "Convenience versus Privacy" tradeoff further in the direction of Convenience.

Space exploration has provided other technoscatological challenges. Venting astronaut urine into space at the wrong times on early missions resulted in a crystalline buildup that fogged capsule windows. Meanwhile, feces proved to be an even stickier problem. For the early, relatively short Mercury missions the men ate low-roughage foods beforehand and simply held it in. For the longer Gemini and Apollo flights, however, NASA gave the crews gloves and adhesive-edged plastic bags. Astronauts taped the bags to their buttocks, helped the feces along with their fingers, wiped, put the paper into the bag, and then added some liquid germicide to the bag before sealing it up and kneading the contents to mix in the germicide. The solution sufficed, but the astronauts hated it. Feces stuck to the buttocks or floated away and stuck to clothes or cabin surfaces, and one astronaut estimated that the entire defecation process typically consumed forty-five minutes!

Meanwhile, since the Vostok programs in the early 60's, the Soviet space program had been using the principle of the vacuum cleaner to collect bodily wastes in zero-g. When NASA designed Skylab, whose longer missions demanded an improvement on plastic bags-preferably something that could also reclaim water—it adopted and expanded upon the Soviet approach. Much developmental effort resulted in the pneumatic Dry John, which sucked cabin air (and feces along with it) through the seat with the spinning vanes and tines of a high-speed "slinger." When the shit literally hit the fan, the slinger shredded it and flung it into a thin layer around the side to dry. A vacuum valve was then opened to draw out water and gases, and the desiccated remainder was stored away for later analysis. Dry John devices succeeded on Skylab and the Space Shuttle, and they're ready for any future staffed interplanetary missions.

On earth, the privately-funded Biosphere 2 project in the Arizona desert tried to address some of the technical problems which may confront long-term human space travel in the future. Biosphere was intended to be a sealed structure containing a mix of species, mostly plants, which could support the lives of its eight-person staff of aging male life sciences professors and nubile young female grad students. While Skylab carried food supplies, the Biosphere approach was to grow the food and fertilize it with excrement in a sustainable cycle. However, high carbon dioxide levels required Biosphere's seal to be broken fairly early in the experiment, indicating that scientists (or at least the scientists involved in the

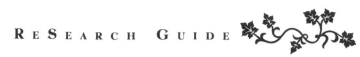

project) still have a great deal to learn about selecting and organizing other species for the purpose of sustaining human life in an artificially closed environment.

Art, Music and Criticism

We're all familiar with the folk parallel between defecating and creating artwork, drawn (for example) in the Cheech and Chong routine in which one dog admires another dog's newly-produced stool with, "Wow, you're a regular Rembrandt! I like the way you put the corn in there for texture!" But in *The Ego Ideal* (1984), Janine Chasseguet-Smirgel suggests that with some artists' creations, the analogy has a literal psychological basis.

Chasseguet-Smirgel outlines two patterns of creativity. The first, based on sublimation of desires (as originally described by Freud in *Civilization and Its Discontents*, 1930), yields art which has the power to short-circuit trains of thought repressed by the viewer, sparking new realizations. The second, based on narcissism, merely carries the message that the viewer is capable of attaining narcissistic fulfillment just like the artist has.

The narcissistic creative pattern originates in childhood, when unhealthy maternal affection leads a boy to believe that he, with his infantile sexuality, is the perfect partner for his mother. As a result, he feels no reason to envy his father and his father's maturity, and his ideal self-image stays halted at a pre-genital state. He idealizes substitutes for the mature penis, beginning with his own feces, which is the first mock-penis he is capable of creating. As he matures, he develops his compulsion to idealize into sophisticated connoisseurship, wherein he fetishizes fake phalluses in the forms of cultural products as well as excrement. Pointing to the sophisticated perversions described by Sade, Chasseguet-Smirgel notes that the narcissistic pervert is, above all, a man of taste. Meanwhile, his deepest fear is that his "secret" might be exposed: that others will realize that his

tastes and play are infantile games and that he merely has a little boy's penis, not the conquering phallus of his fantasies.

In contrast to the authentic art of sublimation, the narcissist's art relies on fakery. He aims to impress with technical virtuosity and intellectual gymnastics, earning from the public the doting admiration his mother once lavished on him. But ultimately, he is merely masking the most mundane content, his own feces, with a dazzling exterior—a process symbolized by a dream remembered by one of Chasseguet-Smirgel's patients. After admitting that he wanted to be a writer, the patient described a dream in which he was taking chocolate logs from a big pile and covering each one with a coat of silver paint, trying not to leave any of the chocolate exposed.

Narcissistic art, Chasseguet-Smirgel explains, frequently achieves the popularity it seeks. The public enjoys illusions, and finds "the fake" fascinating. As an example, she notes a work she saw at a major contemporary art show, a jar of greenish liquid entitled *My Urine in 1962* which she describes as having been "put forward as a 'work' solely by magical virtue of the wish of its author and the complicity of the spectator." While such pieces carry little meaning, they thrill people with the prospect of easily-obtained narcissistic fulfillment.

Chasseguet-Smirgel notes that *My Urine in 1962* plagiarizes works dating back to the time when bodily fluids first entered the Art World, with the Dada movement of the late teens and early twenties. The Dadaists, who were horrified by World War I and viewed it as the inevitable, ultimate expression of bourgeois rationalism, sought to humiliate art and its bourgeois foundation. In 1917, Marcel Duchamp, who led Dada with Jean Arp and others, submitted a urinal, signed (pseudonymously), dated, and titled as a piece of art, for inclusion in the First Annual Exhibition of the Society of Independent Artists in New York. Duchamp himself belonged to the exhibition's jury, but they rejected the piece over his vote, prompting Duchamp to resign and exhibit the urinal elsewhere. *Fountain*, as the piece was called, has been lost, but a photograph of it by Alfred

Steiglitz is reproduced in many art textbooks. It remains one of the century's most influential works.

Another Duchamp creation, from 1919, consisted of a color reproduction of the Mona Lisa with a mustache and beard penciled in. Its title, *L.H.O.O.Q.*, spoken quickly, sounds like the sentence "she has a hot ass" in French ("Elle a chaud au cul").

Meanwhile, in Berlin, Richard Huelsenbeck and John Heartfield rallied the local Dada scene with the call and response, "What is German Culture? Shit!" Huelsenbeck put a characteristic inter-war German spin on the aspirations of Dada by proposing to destroy revered values with "all the instruments of satire, bluff, irony, and, finally, violence. . .in a great common action." Berlin's Dada scene climaxed in 1920 when it hosted the International Dada Fair, the central symbol of which was a uniformed German officer with the head of a pig.

During the mid-twenties, Dada merged with the next artistic current, Surrealism. The most prominent surrealist, Salvador Dali, was fascinated by excrement. He discussed it frequently and depicted it in many of his paintings, demonstrating that, as he once wrote, "the excrementitious palette enjoys infinite variety, from gray to green and from ochers to browns."

The first Dali painting to contain blatant scatology, *Lugubrious Game* (1929 depicts in its foreground a man wearing shit-stained underwear. André Breton, Surrealism's leading theorist, was appalled. However, in an essay about the painting, Georges Bataille, a contemporary of Breton's, associated the stain with the rediscovery of virility. Where Breton rejected scatology, Bataille embraced it. In "The Solar Anus," Bataille describes interactions between celestial bodies, global features and life forms as giant acts of coitus and defecation. In "The Jesuve" and "The Pineal Eye," Bataille remarks on the brightly-colored protruding anuses of many tree-dwelling primates and traces their diminution, following the disappearance of the tail in the course of human evolution. He imagines a new version of this primate

anus, the "Pineal Eye," bursting out of the tops of our heads, re-emerging from the new seat of our equilibrium. These essays and others address sexuality, scatology, mortality, and other aspects of human animality which threatened prevailing rationalistic belief systems. Bataille influenced contemporary theorists such as Jacques Derrida, Michel Foucault and Jean Baudrillard.

In Zygmunt Bauman's "The sweet scent of decomposition," from *Forget Baudrillard?* (1993), a book of commentary on Baudrillard (the title of which is an insiders reference to "Forget Foucault," a Baudrillard critique of Foucault), Bauman notes Baudrillard's frequent references to shit, sex, and death in his writing, and his heavy use of olfactory and tactile metaphors, and shows how this postmodernist sensibility clashes with modernity, which futilely tried to extinguish smells because they reminded modernists of their failure to control living processes and to overcome death. Modernity attempted to eclipse contemplation of death with a series of short-lived fashions, revivals, and revivals of revivals to instill the notion that no loss is truly permanent. In contrast, the po-mo approach to mortality, in my reading of Bauman's essay, seems to lie somewhere in between "To life, to life, L'Chiam" and "Oh well, whatever, never mind . . . ."

As Tom Wolfe suggests, the line between Art and Criticism seems to have disappeared. Now insider artists and critics operate in concert, stroking each other to mutually build up their stature before their own eyes and the eyes of the public. You can see the inevitable result in the paintings of Mark Tansey, which depict monumental, heroic edifices built out of deconstructionist texts and portray relatively recent art world occurrences posited by critics as pivotal moments in world history. Not all artists depict criticism as reverently as Tansey does, however. One example is the drawing "Satire On Art Criticism," which shows a group of men gathered around a painting. One of them has the upright ears of an ass, and wears a serious expression on his face as he talks and gestures toward the painting with his pipe. All but one of the rest of the men listen intently. The remaining one

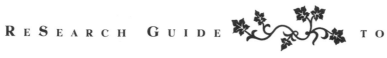

squats next to the painting, pants down, wiping himself after having just defecated. The artist of the drawing, Rembrandt, sketched the scene with just enough detail to get his point across, but he signed it carefully and prominently.

Since the days of Dada and Surrealism, artists have continued to use references to bodily functions as a tried and true formula for shocking the bourgeoisie and pledging allegiance to the side of Free Expression. One well-known recent example, which relies on obvious sacrilege, is Andres Serrano's *Piss Christ* (1987), a crucifix immersed in urine, which stood at the center of a recent dispute regarding government funding of art. A slightly more subtle approach involves tricking the viewer into realizing (after some examination) that an aesthetically pleasing artwork has scatological origins. This was achieved by Wim Delvoye's tiled entrance floor for 1992's Documenta IX international art exhibition in Kassel, Germany. The "abstract" patterns had been inspired by the artist's stools!

A few artists bring more complexity into scatological works, taking them beyond simple flag-waving. An untitled work (1987-1990) by Kiki Smith, for example, consists of a row of twelve glass carboys, each labeled, in the Fraktur script of a medieval German alchemist, with the name of a different liquid our bodies produce: urine, tears, blood, semen, mucus, saliva, diarrhea, oil, vomit, sweat, milk, and pus. A metallic finish prevents us from seeing into the bottles, reflecting our gazes back at ourselves. Another sculpture by Smith, *Tale* (1992) portrays a woman crawling along the ground as if cursed like the serpent in Eden, with a long turd emerging from her anus and trailing behind her.

Artists have also referred to Duchamp more literally by representing the fixtures associated with elimination rather than the products themselves. Examples are Claes Oldenburg's *Soft Toilet* and *Ghost Toilet*, and Paul McCarthy's toilet stall partitions from the Los Angeles MOCA's 1992 "Helter Skelter" exhibit.

For a while, the Art World didn't know exactly what to make of another sanitary fixture, an ac-

tual, working three-hole wooden outhouse seat painted in the style of Jackson Pollock by Willem de Kooning (possibly with the help of Pollock himself, who was one of his roommates at the time) during the summer of 1954, while de Kooning, Pollock, and others were sharing a house on Long Island. A nearby auctioneer bought the seat for fifty dollars in the mid-eighties, and it was scheduled for auction at Sotheby's in February 1992.

Before the auction, opinions on the seat's worth varied widely. Some thought it should be valued as highly as any other early de Kooning—possibly more so, owing to its uniqueness. Others, such as Arthur C. Danto, disagreed. In *The Nation*, Danto rationalized that the seat did not fit in with de Kooning's work at the time: "Its mock Pollockian marbling is isolated from everything that went before and came after." Therefore it is a mere artifact, rather than true art. Duchamp's *Fountain*, on the other hand, which de Kooning's seat had been compared to, fit in with the issues Duchamp was exploring at the time. Danto did admit, nevertheless, that the outhouse seat "has some archaeological significance as a reminder of *la vie de bohème* led by artists near Amagansett before they all became famous."

Pre-auction appraisals of the object reflected the split opinion, ranging from ten thousand to over one million dollars. Unfortunately, the piece was withdrawn from auction, so its value as art remains a mystery.

Underground comics portray bodily functions so frequently, it's almost a genre requirement. In the late Sixties, the first underground comics began distinguishing themselves from mainstream sequential art through scatology as well as slang, realism, anti-establishment attitudes, and references to sex, drugs, and rock 'n' roll. Today, underground comics are more scatological than ever. Recent examples include Chester Brown's *Ed the Happy Clown*, in which an unsuspecting man's prolific anus turns out to be a portal to another universe, and Julie Doucet's "Heavy Flow," from *Weirdo #26*, which caricatures the travail of getting your period and not having any tampons in the house. Other Rabelaisian cartoonists include Robert Crumb, Sam Gross, Joe Matt, and Gilbert Shelton. Similarly, the animated television cartoon *The Ren & Stimpy Show*, directed by John Kricfalusi, was jam-packed with bathroom antics.

Of all branches of art, though, Performance has in recent years been associated most closely with bodily functions, perhaps because the medium lends itself so well to shock, the usual raison d'être. Genuine excrement and excretory acts taken out of their proper places and offered as art repulse more strongly and violate more taboos than mere representations.

The Aktionist movement in Vienna during the late sixties staged many such pieces. One event took place at the University of Vienna in 1969. A young man walked onto the stage, removed his clothing, urinated into his cupped hands, drank the urine, and then vomited. Then, for his finale, he turned around, defecated, and smeared the shit all over his body while singing the Austrian national anthem.

In *We Keep Our Victims Ready* (1991), Karen Finley suggested the same sort of dramatic finale by smearing herself with chocolate frosting while reciting a text about the difficulties of love and the aggressive nature of men. In other pieces, Finley has employed yams as well as frosting to symbolize feces.

The Los Angeles based dance troupe Contraband performs a modern version of a coming of age ritual in which audience members spit into a bowl. The performers then add food coloring to the communal saliva and smear themselves with it. They also smear themselves with blood let from veins in their own legs.

In *Tubes* (1991), the members of Blue Man Group appear to excrete a processed-cheese-like substance from orifices in the middles of their chests, which they then divide among themselves and eat.

But the most notorious excremental performer of recent years came out of punk rock, not performance art. Before succumbing to heroin in 1993, G. G. Allin, of G. G. Allin and the Scumfuks, kept his audiences awake by shitting

diarrhea on stage (he took laxatives before performances), flinging it at the audience, putting it in his mouth, spitting it into the audience, and engaging in other similar antics. Other rockers have integrated excremental horseplay into their performances as well, though not as forcefully as Allin. John Lydon sodomized himself with a banana. Mike Patton of Mr. Bungle gave himself an enema.

As with sequential and performance art, music has only recently started to refer to bodily functions with any frequency. Mozart wrote a couple of short vocal pieces around the text "Lick my ass," and Richard Strauss used the contrabassoon to portray loss of bowel control in his tone poem *Till Eulenspiegel's Merry Pranks* (1895). During World War II, the Spike Jones Orchestra punctuated their hit "In Der Führer's Face" with a "raspberry" after each "Heil" in the refrain. Screamin' Jay Hawkins brought an earthy, mock-voodoo sensibility to his music during the fifties, and still performs his "Constipation Blues" as an encore. During the sixties, The Fugs and Frank Zappa began mining the territory as well. But it wasn't until the eighties' rise of suburban punk and rap that scatology became widespread in underground music.

Today, it's almost a requirement for punk/alternative/garage/underground rock bands to write songs about excretions, or even invoke them with their names. Old timers who lament that youngsters today don't value wordplay in music as they did in the days of Noel Coward and Cole Porter need only look to band names such as Anus the Menace, Pat Smear, Public Enema and Archers of Loaf to see that verbal cleverness is alive and well.

Good recent examples of excretory references in music include the EP *Anal By Anal* (reissued 1993) by Boredoms, featuring songs such as "Anal Eat," "God From Anal," and "Born to Anal," the bathroom ballad "The Toilet's Flooded," from *Stinky Grooves* (1990) by Limbomaniacs, and Biz Markie's "Pickin' Boogers," from *Goin' Off* (1988), and "Toilet Stool Rap," from *I Need A Haircut* (1991).

At least one scribe for the "alternative" press was put off enough by "Pickin' Boogers" to write, "*Goin' Off* is a dubious debut, opening with a supremely obnoxious ode to something too tasteless to go into." The censorious review appeared in the *Trouser Press Record Guide* (4th edition), subtitled "The Ultimate Guide to Alternative Music." The oft-requested video for "Toilet Stool Rap," meanwhile, was banned by MTV, BET, and Video Jukebox Network, but managed to reach receptive audiences on locally-produced video shows. The *Village Voice* named the "Toilet Stool Rap" video one of the year's ten best.

Folklore

Self-conscious "high" culture may snub the scatological, but throughout the world, folklore embraces it in myths, superstitions, jokes, and sayings.

Many creation myths explain that the land, the seas, and the first people originated as the feces and urine of the gods. The Siberian god Raven created land by crapping while flying over the earth's waters. For Kodiak Islanders, the land came first, and the oceans spread from the urine of the first woman. Similarly, Australian natives attribute the oceans to the time that Pund-jel, angered by people's wickedness, tried to drown the entire world with his urine. More recently, European friars embellished our own deluge myth by explaining that initially during the Flood, Noah put all the animals' dung behind a bulkhead astern the Ark, but when it started weighing too much, they threw it all overboard, creating the Americas.

Many myths explain ordinary rain as the urine of gods, such as the Kamchatkan myth that Billutschi produces the rain when he pees, and when he is done, he puts on a new dress with fringes of red seal hair and colored leather, making the rainbow.

The anthropology and folklore literature that recounts the world's myths profiles a variety of earthy characters, including Excrement Woman, Dung-Being, Diarrhea-Man, and Snot Boy. Many of the scatological stories, such as the British Columbian Eskimo legend of Grass-Woman and Diarrhea-Man, reflect male jealousy of procreative power and the resulting fantasy of giving birth through the anus.

Other stories show no such yearning, such as the Kamchatkan tale of the foolish god Kutka, who falls in love with his own feces, woos it as his bride, takes it home in his sleigh, and only realizes his mistake after he takes it into his bed.

Myths often ascribe magical properties to excrement. The Hindu god Utanka became immortal by eating bull dung. Discovering the droppings of the Guinean god of the rainbow, the serpent Aidowedo, imparts the ability to turn grain kernels into money. Many folktales also associate feces with wealth. The European story of The Goose That Laid the Golden Egg may have started out as one such tale.

Superstitions also connect logs with lucre, and, more generally, good luck. According to a rural French superstition, stepping in dung presages coming into money. Both Germans and Italians believed that being hit with a bird-dropping bodes well. During the 17th Century, Dutch prostitutes sought to bring luck to their houses by putting fresh horse dung by the front door.

Excrement from both animals and humans has been used worldwide to divine the future, ward off evil, and cast hexes. Australian aborigines buried their feces to prevent it from falling into enemy hands. Europeans believed that human feces would ward off evil because the Devil hated it. They also fought perceived evils with urine; in Minden, Germany, boys would cross their urine streams and incant, "Kreuspissen, morgen stirbst ein Jude" (Piss criss-cross, tomorrow a Jew will die).

Many folk love potions and aphrodisiacs contain human and animal excrement, as do many love potion antidotes and anti-aphrodisiacs. Traditional fertility charms also frequently contain feces.

Cures and spells can require other body products as well. A French cure from the late 1600's instructed a man to tie his nail clippings to the back of a living crab, throw it into a stream, and then return home without speaking. A rickets cure from New England consisted of burying a lock of the afflicted child's hair at a crossroads during a full moon.

These superstitions usually grow out of belief in sympathetic magic, which seems to occur in all cultures. Early science carried over these beliefs, as evidenced by a treatise on "Magnetism" from 1801 which recommends that if a prankster takes a dump at your door, you should poke it with a red-hot poker and thereby, through "Magnetism" (a "scientific" recasting of sympathetic magic beliefs), inflame the offender's anus.

Plenty of sayings owe their popularity to the strength of scatological imagery. In his study of German culture, *Life Is Like A Chicken Coop Ladder*, folklorist Alan Dundes offers numerous examples. One such proverb, "Life is like a chicken coop ladder—short and shitty," which has several variants, provided the study's title. Dundes also notes "The more beautiful the cow, the larger the cowflop," and "Good shitting can be lots of fun/Sometimes much more tha+n fucking someone." Other earthy folk aphorisms are somewhat less clear, such as "No cow shits exactly one pound," also noted by Dundes, and "The more you cry, the less you piss," from Bourke.

Some folk riddles also focus on excretions, such as the traditional Kamchatkan riddle about human feces:

My father has numerous forms and dresses; my mother is warm and thin and bears every day. Before I am born, I like cold and warmth, but after I am born, only cold. In the cold I am strong, and in the warmth, weak; if cold, I am seen far; if warm, I am smelled far.

Like any other taboo-repression area, bodily functions inspire more than their share of jokes. One representative example of bathroom humor recounts an exchange in a men's room between a C.I.A. man and an F.B.I. man. Both have just used the urinals. As the F.B.I. man walks to the door, the C.I.A. man walks to the sink, turns on the faucet, and says, "In the C.I.A., we always wash our hands after we relieve ourselves." Walking out the door, the F.B.I. man replies, "In the F.B.I., we don't 'relieve ourselves' on our fingers." Variations of the joke substitute other rival organizations, such as Harvard and Yale, or the Army and the Navy.

Urban legends, like jokes, are another familiar modern form of folklore. One bawdy example recounts the story of a drunken lacrosse player at a victory party who invites a babe at the party to join him upstairs. She accepts and the two walk up to his room. They start making out, and in the course of human events, the babe asks the dude to make love to her. The two undress, but when the dude starts putting on a condom, a wave of nausea hits him. He vomits huge amounts all over the babe and then passes out. The next morning, he wakes up with a wicked hangover. The babe has left, but he finds a massive turd on his chest, with a note on it that reads, "I hope you know how pissed off I was to actually shit on you . . . ."

Because they're often written in bathrooms, graffiti may be the most frequently scatological of all branches of folklore. One classier-than-usual example, from a men's room in London's Parliament building, reads:

"In the House up above, when a motion is read,
The Member stands up and uncovers his head;
In this House down below, when a motion's to pass,
The Member sits down. . ."

You can find more jokes, urban legends, and graffiti in collections such as the *Truly Tasteless Jokes* series, by "Blanche Knott," *The Vanishing Hitchhiker*, *The Mexican Pet*, and *The Choking Doberman*, by Jan Harold Brunvand, and *Graffiti: Two Thousand Years of Wall Writing* and *The Encyclopedia of Graffiti*, by Robert G. Reisner.

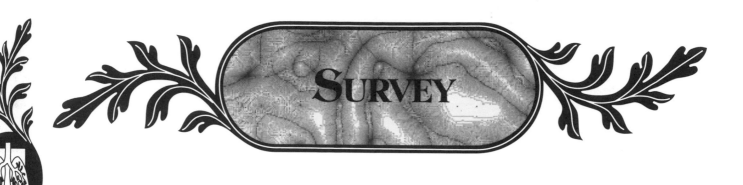

Survey Methodology

A total of 106 people, 66 men and 40 women, filled out my questionnaire, the final version which we have reprinted here. The men ranged from 17 to 48 years of age, with a median age of 25, an average age of 26.24, and a standard deviation of 7.123 years. The more compact womens' sample ranged from 16 to 39 with a standard deviation of 5.059 years, a median age of 19.5 and a mean of 21.85. In both cases, respondents' ages clustered around just below the median ages, with a handful of outliers in their thirties and forties pulling the mean up.

Participants came from three sources: the Internet, friends of mine, and people on the U.C. Berkeley campus. I distributed and received fourteen of the questionnaires through the Internet, posting a query to the newsgroup *rec.humor* in the Spring of 1990 and posting the questionnaire itself to the newsgroup *alt.tasteless* in the Spring of 1991. I received six completed questionnnaires from *rec.humor* readers and eight from the *alt.tasteless* readers. All but one of the fourteen of these were men, and most were either computer professionals or students of Computer Science.

I printed and distributed the rest of the questionnaires by hand. Of these 92 hardcopy versions, 21 were filled out by friends and aquaintances of mine during the Spring of 1990 and 47 and 24 of them respectively were filled out on two sunny afternoons in the summer and fall of 1991 by people in Sproul Plaza on the campus of the University of California at Berkeley who responded favorably to my repeated cries of "Fill out a questionnaire for a dollar! Make an easy buck; fill out a questionnaire!"

(In addition to the total of 106 mentioned, I also received fourteen completed questionnaires at the American Booksellers Association convention in 1994. These I culled for word answers only, not including them in any of the statistics.)

I won't argue that the 106 people queried represent a cross-section of the American public, but I do feel my survey represents young adult America at least as well as any in the grand tradition of Psychology studies that conclude universals from the behavior of undergrad Psych majors fulfilling their one-credit Study Participation requirements.

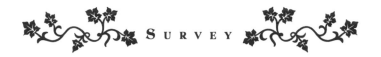

Bodily Fluids Survey Questionnaire

Please feel free to:

Answer only some of the questions.

Digress and discuss interesting relevant points or relate amusing anecdotes. (Write them on the back).

Briefly describe yourself (age, sex, occupation, etc.).

In general, how do you feel about bodily functions such as mucus production, urination, and defecation? Do you feel that most others share your views?

Nasal Hygiene

Where, typically, do you pick your nose (bathroom, car, kitchen . . .)?

What do you do with the "boogers" once you've snagged them?

Ever give yourself a nosebleed from excessively vigorous picking?

Would you say you "enjoy" picking your nose?

If so, do you do ever do anything to ensure that there'll be plenty to pick (hike dusty trails, snort breadcrumbs . . .)?

Ever picked anyone else's nose? Whose? How old were you?

Ever place objects in your nostrils (coins, marbles . . .)? Ever "lose" anything up there? How did you finally get it out (if you ever did, that is)?

Did you ever deposit a booger someplace you wish you hadn't? Where might that have been?

Do you like the actor Slim Pickens?

Do you blow your nose? What are some unusual things you've blown your nose into when you haven't had a tissue or hanky?

Ever blow your nose into "thin air"? Where did it land? Ever blow your nose in the shower?

Do you ever sneeze gobs of mucus onto your hand? What do you do with them if you don't have a hanky handy?

Vomiting

When was the last time you threw up?

What were the surrounding circumstances?

Do you throw up often? About how often?

Have you ever made yourself throw up? Why?

What was the most embarrassing place you ever threw up?

Ever "chug" and then "power boot"? How far did it go? Did you win? Who did?

What is your favorite food to throw up (if such a preference has ever occurred to you)?

Ever make anyone else throw up? How? Why?

Urination

Do you get "Asparagus pee"? "Coffee pee"? "Neon Multivitamin pee"?

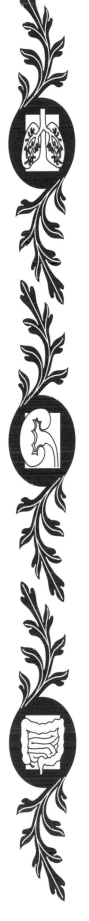

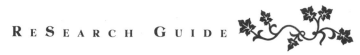

Ever time your pees? What's your "record"? Ever break a minute without beer?

Do you pee in the shower?

(Guys:) Ever pee out the window of a moving car?
(Gals:) Ever accidentally pee a little from laughing too much?

Ever pee while in a swimming pool? Public or private? Was this recent? How about in a hot tub? No way!

(Gals:) Ever use the men's room because the line was too long for the women's and it was an "emergency"?
(Guys:) Ever find it hard to pee if there's a long line of people waiting behind you? Ever use a toilet stall purely for privacy's sake?

Do you sometimes briefly shiver in the middle of a long pee?

(Guys:) How do you pee with an early morning erection? Or do you just wait?

Where do you like to pee outdoors? Have you ever peed from the top of a tree? Off a cliff?

(Guys:) Do you use the fly on undies, do you pull them down, or do you pull one of the leg holes up and around? Do you favor boxers or briefs?

(Guys:) Do you usually flush urinals? If not, why not?

Defecation

Ever pinch a loaf so big that part of it stuck out of the water?

Ever wipe with leaves? Dirt? Your hand? Paper money?

Do you crumple your toilet paper or fold it?

About how many squares do you tear off at once? About how many wipes do get per tear? About how many tears will take care of your average loaf?

Do you wipe front to back (i.e. bottom to top), back to front, or just back and forth? Do you reach around behind your back or reach back through between your legs?

Do you look at the paper after a wipe?

Do you stand to wipe or remain seated and lean over?

Do you like to watch it go down after a flush?

Ever moisten the paper for improved cleaning ability? How?

Does eating highly spiced foods affect your loaves the next day?

Does drinking coffee help give you "the urge"? Smoking a cigarette?

Would you consider yourself "regular"? How many loaves do you pinch per day? At what times?

Ever see kernels of corn in your loaves? Peanuts? Tomato seeds? Other distinguishable objects?

Do you eat breakfast cereal? A high-fiber variety? Are you pleased with its effect on your stool?

Do you ever avoid any food or any class of food because you don't like the effect it has on your loaves?

Are you reluctant to pinch a loaf away from home? What's the most uncomfortable place you've ever had to pinch a loaf?

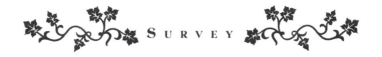

Do you fear "toilet water splash-back"? Do you like it?

Are you a world traveller? How have you found foreign types of toilets to be?

What's your "record" for how long you've gone without pinching a loaf? Were you travelling then?

Flatus Expulsion

About how many times per day do you usually fart?

What foods do you associate with flatulence (besides the obvious ones)?

In what social situations do you allow yourself to fart? In situations in which you hold it back, when do you finally let it go (bathroom visit, outside, end of evening, crowded dance floor . . .)? Do you generally excuse yourself or otherwise say anything to acknowledge it? What do you say?

(Singles:) How long (if at all) do you have to be "going out" with someone before you'll fart in their company? Do you just wait for them to go first? How long do they typically take?

(Marrieds:) Do you fart freely in the presence of your spouse when there's just the two of you there?

Ever ignite a fart? What color did it glow? Did you singe any hairs?

Ever fart onto your hand? Did you sniff your hand afterwards? Were you at all surprised? Do you think this is sick behavior?

Ever fart while swimming? Were you wearing a skin-tight bathing suit? A wetsuit? Did anyone comment, or did they just pretend not to notice?

Ever "blame" someone else for one of your farts? Ever been in a situation in which everyone comments, but no one admits responsibilty? Was it in a car?

Are there any related questions you think I should have asked? What are they?

Thank you very much for your candid participation.

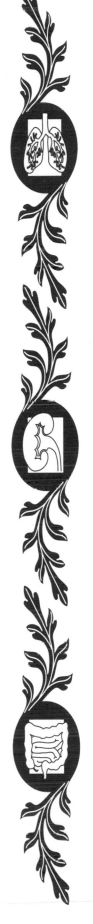

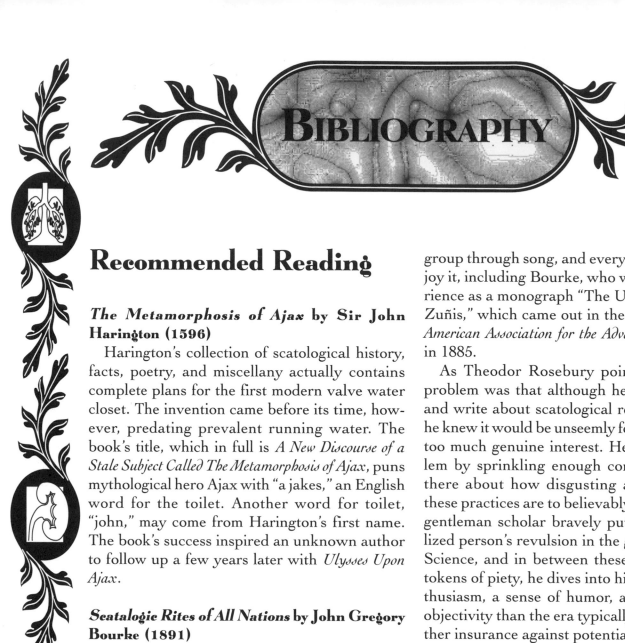

Recommended Reading

The Metamorphosis of Ajax by Sir John Harington (1596)

Harington's collection of scatological history, facts, poetry, and miscellany actually contains complete plans for the first modern valve water closet. The invention came before its time, however, predating prevalent running water. The book's title, which in full is *A New Discourse of a Stale Subject Called The Metamorphosis of Ajax*, puns mythological hero Ajax with "a jakes," an English word for the toilet. Another word for toilet, "john," may come from Harington's first name. The book's success inspired an unknown author to follow up a few years later with *Ulysses Upon Ajax*.

Scatalogic Rites of All Nations by John Gregory Bourke (1891)

After years of research, John G. Bourke, U.S. Army cavalry captain and anthropologist (translation: expert in Native American peoples and how to exterminate them), published this 496-page dissertation on the roles of excrement in religion, medicine, and daily life throughout the world. The event which inspired Captain Bourke to embark upon this immense task occurred ten years earlier, on November 17th, 1881.

That night, Captain Bourke, staying with fellow anthropologist Frank Cushing in New Mexico, attended a Zuñi medicine dance. There he saw dancers urinate into pails and then drink each others' urine, and one Zuñi mentioned that had the dance been performed outdoors, they would have consumed feces as well. The ceremony also included carousing, clowning around, and lampooning different personalities in the group through song, and everyone seemed to enjoy it, including Bourke, who wrote up the experience as a monograph "The Urine Dance of the Zuñis," which came out in the *Transactions of the American Association for the Advancement of Science* in 1885.

As Theodor Rosebury points out, Bourke's problem was that although he wanted to study and write about scatological religious practices, he knew it would be unseemly for his tone to show too much genuine interest. He solves the problem by sprinkling enough comments here and there about how disgusting and un-Christian these practices are to believably play the role of a gentleman scholar bravely putting aside a civilized person's revulsion in the greater interest of Science, and in between these tongue in cheek tokens of piety, he dives into his subject with enthusiasm, a sense of humor, and more genuine objectivity than the era typically allowed. As further insurance against potential objections to his study, Bourke's title page prominently warns, "Not For General Perusal."

The work focuses on religious rites, but because cultures' world views often tie religion in with what we would call medicine, custom, folklore, crafts, and industry, it's really a cross cultural survey of scatology in all aspects of life. *Scatalogic Rites* provided much of the information in Chapter 6: *All Excreta*.

None other than Sigmund Freud wrote the foreword to the 1913 German translation of *Scatalogic Rites*.

The Specialist by Chic Sale (1929)

This short book came out of a popular character monologue 45-year-old stage actor and comedian Charles "Chic" Sale had been performing at Rotary Club functions and in vaudeville shows across the country. Sale based the monologue on a carpenter he knew from his home town of Urbana, Illinois who specialized in building outhouses and who knew well all the considerations good outhouse design entailed. Its warm, nostalgic, down-home humor must have presented urbane Twenties audiences and readers with the same sort of appeal Garrison Keillor, Bill Franzen, Tom Bodett, and others engender today, and by word-of-mouth alone (no advertising), the thin volume soon became a runaway bestseller, moving a million copies within a couple of years. The craze for *The Specialist* capped a golden age for scatological humor in this country, prompting Stanley Walker to write, in 1935, "It is a toss-up whether the bed or the bathroom is more significant in American humor." The expression "chic sale" even entered the language as slang for outhouse, much to the author's chagrin. (Sale came to view the book's popularity as a mixed blessing—for the rest of his life, his name was associated with outhouses. He died in 1936, before managing to broaden his reputation with successes involving other topics.) To date, *The Specialist* has sold over two and a half million copies, and it is still available from Specialist Publishing Company in Burlingame, California, which sells Sale's also-quite-funny 1930 sequel, *I'll Tell You Why*.

Through the Alimentary Canal With a Gun and a Camera by George S. Chappell (1930)

In 1911, Robert Benchley, old master of American Humor, was a wacky college boy at Harvard displaying his talent for literate irreverence by giving parody lectures every few weeks in Harvard's Arnold Arboretum after hours, when the Arboretum was supposed to be closed. Benchley's "lectures," with names like "The Affinity of Dogs for Dogwood, on the Basis of Natural Selection," and "Beards, their Rise and Fall, Use and Abuse," got to be more and more popular, until one time when he whipped the crowd into such a frenzy that they marched en masse out to the yard behind the Administration building and lit a bonfire so big that it visibly scorched some of the University's beloved slippery-elms. As a result of instigating this unauthorized bonfire Benchley was kicked out of the Arnold Arboretum permanently. The title of this inflammatory lecture was "Through the Alimentary Canal With a Gun and a Camera." George Chappell, a Yale man ten years Benchley's senior, was in attendance and it became such a fond memory for him that twenty years later, when both Chappell and Benchley were firmly established, *New Yorker* affiliated humorists, Chappell decided to expand on Benchley's idea and turn *Through the Alimentary Canal . . .* into a book.

Satirizing the era's popular adventure travel genre, *Through the Alimentary Canal . . .* describes the perilous journey two gentlemen-explorers undertake to the interior of a man's abdomen. Among other exotic adventures, the intrepid pair explore the Oral Cavern and the Nerve Forest of the Lumbar Region, find the Source of the Bile, boat down the Upper and Lower Colon, meet with His Excellency, the Duodenum at his estate in Pylorus, and visit the Appendix (although, as Duodenum notes, it isn't nearly as impressive as it used to be). The book was published in 1930 with an introduction by Benchley (whom Chappell calls "The Columbus of the Colon") and illustrations by *New Yorker* cartoonist Otto Soglow with titles like "I Land My First Phagocyte" and "He Insisted on Carving His Initials on the Spinal Column."

Cleanliness And Godliness by Reginald Reynolds (1943)

Reynolds greatly admired Sir John Harington's *The Metamorphosis Of Ajax*, and saw his own work as a knock-off. Of Harington's work he writes, "it is my hope that by drawing so much attention to this work I may arouse some publisher, such as my friend Mr. Unwin, to bring out this book of Sir John's once more, though I know well enough that it will put my own to shame."

Reynolds began writing to escape the tension and horror of London life during World War II. His book is a freely-connecting and highly personal work (i.e. borderline insane rambling—but in a good way) that visits such topics as the history of toilets and toilet paper, the history of personal hygiene, scatological proverbs, bathroom

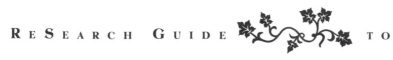

graffiti, and organic farming.

The book becomes more focused toward the end when it begins to discuss organic farming. Reynolds argues that sewage should be used as fertilizer instead of being piped into the sea, suggesting a cyclical truck route of produce to cities and sewage back to farms. He discusses the successful use of sewage sludge as fertilizer in experimental communities and by regular farmers. The new enemies of the environment, Reynolds asserts, are sterility and the chemical fertilizer companies. On the last page he concludes, "I began this book to escape from a world that wearied me, and believing that the best part of Man went down the drain; but I have come back through space and eternity to expose one of the worst *rackets* in the world, by which I mean the trade in chemical fertilizers."

Life Against Death by Norman O. Brown (1959)

In this book, Professor Brown, who helped build up the intellectual underpinnings for the youth movement of the Sixties and whose 1960 speech to the Columbia University chapter of Phi Beta Kappa (reprinted in May 1961's *Harper's*) is viewed by some as the movement's inaugural address, psychoanalyzes our history in Freudian terms and explains the high cost repression has had on our society and the higher costs it will have if we insist on clinging to it in the future. The book's later chapters diagnose our culture's anality and discuss excrement's threat to our repressed outlook, as recognized by Freud and, before him, Jonathan Swift.

Life On Man by Theodor Rosebury (1969)

Microbiologist Rosebury makes a strong and eloquent case for abandoning our obsession with germs, cleanliness, and deodorization. He begins by breaking the news to us that our bodies and our world are filled with microbes that enable our own and all life's survival. He then traces the historical origins and evolution of our taboos and prejudices against excrement and sex from early Judaism through Christianity and literature and

into our present culture and shows how, after Pasteur and Koch's germ theory, the old superstitions remained with the public, but with a new name for the filthy evil spirits: germs.

Today, consumer products manufacturers profit by spreading and reinforcing these beliefs under the guise of science, and so despite the medical understanding that most microbes in and on us are innocuous or beneficial and that infection by potentially harmful ones usually requires much more than casual exposure, the compulsively neat, anal public spends unhealthy amounts of time, money, and mental energy on antiseptics, antiperspirants, etc. Dr. Rosebury concludes by asking where the genuine obscenities in our culture lie: "Is it the healthy body, its parts, functions, and products, or the exhalations of automobiles and smokestacks? . . . . Is it the 'obscenities' hurled by unarmed civilians, or the swinging nightsticks and billowing nausea gas of helmeted and masked police? Is it normal microbes or perverted men?"

The Bathroom (second edition) by Alexander Kira (1976)

The first edition of this book came out in 1966 as a part of a large research report by Cornell's Center For Housing and Environmental Design. Professor Kira's domain on the project was to study and define criteria for the design of the modern bathroom. His groundbreaking report immediately became an ergonomics landmark, and its enormous popularity led him to revise and expand it considerably and publish the resulting second edition commercially.

In writing the books, architect Kira studied anatomy, social history, psychology, and many other fields, took photographs, made measurements, drew up plans, built mock-ups, and ran experiments. He concludes that we would do well to substantially change our bathrooms and bathroom fixtures, and provides improved designs and layouts to help enact such a change. For example, finding dry paper wiping suboptimal for cleansing and sitting upright worse for defecation than squatting, Kira proposes designs with footrests and leg supports for a more squat-like posture and water spouts for better cleansing options. Kira also shows how to modify existing toilets for greater comfort, including add-on footrests and an improved seat. Leaving no factor of use unexamined, Kira provides bathroom floor plans and suggestions and designs for sinks, showers, urinals, bidets, and bathtubs as well as for toilets.

End Product: The First Taboo by Dan Sabbath (1977)

When self-titled "anthroscatologist" Dan Sabbath was writing this beautiful and clever paean to feces, he notes, whenever anyone around him mentioned shit, everyone in the room would look his way. Sabbath brings history, science, and current events into his discussion, but draws most of all on his own mastery of the language and sense of humor. Like Reynolds, Sabbath concludes his book with a plug for organic farming.

Histoire de la Merde (Prologue) by Dominique Laporte (1978)

If you're interested in scatology and know French, you would undoubtedly enjoy this book. I don't know French, unfortunately, so I can't tell you anything more about it.

Toilet Learning by Alison Mack (1978)

Toilet Learning is a potty-training manual published, appropriately enough, by Little, Brown and Company. The book is divided into two sections, one for parents and one for children. The children's section is a picture-book for parents to read through with their kids to explain the basics. Excerpt: "One of the things that comes out of you is wet./We call it wee-wee./See the rain puddle?/Rain is wet." I would imagine that the section works well, although its depictions of bell-bottoms, afros, earth shoes, and embroidery may not ring true for more fashion-aware toddlers. The parents' section not only provides a page-by-page instructional commentary on the children's section, but also details the evolution of potty-training theory and practice throughout the century, quoting past generations' child care books as well

as Sigmund Freud and Erik Erikson.

Life Is Like A Chicken Coop Ladder by Alan Dundes (1984)

Taking its title from a German folk one-liner ("Life is like a chicken coop ladder—short and shitty"), this book elaborates on the controversial presidential address Professor Dundes presented at the 1980 meeting of the American Folklore Society, an address which angered some folklorists yet prompted another to call it a "turd de force." Dundes's argues that "national character" is a meaningful concept that can be seen, for example, in the German's special interest in the scatological, and in supporting his thesis he takes a fascinating tour through German folklore, literature, art, and history, showing links and shared themes among all of them and contrasting them to those of other cultures.

The Foul and the Fragrant by Alain Corbin (1986), originally published as Le Miasme et la Jonquille (1982)

Subtitled *Odor and the French Social Imagination*, this book examines the historical significance of the sense of smell during and following one of smell's most important eras, the late 1700's in France, which saw "perceptual revolution" as well as political revolution. It's interesting to follow how smell acquired scientific and social importance, changing a society of ubiquitous, unquestioned, and unopposed stink into one which controlled its olfactory environment and read odors as signs of health, social status, personal identity, and sensuality. Plus, the old descriptions of how disgusting Paris was on the eve of the Revolution are amazing.

The Vanishing American Outhouse by Ronald S. Barlow (1989)

Antiquarian Barlow has brought together history, folklore, old Government pamphlets, plans, and nearly two hundred photographs of privies and related objects into one big coffee-table-suitable browsing book.

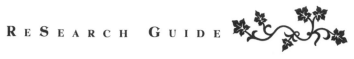

Bibliography

Report of the Surgeon General's Workshop on Breastfeeding and Human Lactation. Rockville, Maryland: U. S. Department of Health and Human Services, 1984.

Ackerman, Diane. *A Natural History of the Senses*. New York: Random House, Inc., 1990.

Adams, Cecil. *More of The Straight Dope*. New York: Ballantine Books, 1988.

Adams, Cecil. *The Straight Dope*. New York: Ballantine Books, 1986.

Afonsky, D. *Saliva and its Relation to Oral Health*. University, Alabama: University of Alabama Press, 1961.

Agee, James and Walker Evans. *Let Us Now Praise Famous Men*. New York: Houghton Mifflin Company, 1941.

Alpers, Svetlana. *Rembrandt's Enterprise*. Chicago: The University of Chicago Press, 1988.

Barbieri, Robert. "Etiology and Epidemiology of Endometriosis," *The American Journal of Obstetrics and Gynecology* vol. 162, no. 2. St. Louis: The C. V. Mosby Company, February 1990.

Barlow, Ronald S. *The Vanishing American Outhouse*. El Cajon, California: Windmill Publishing Company, 1989.

Barnes, Richard H. "Nutritional Implications of Coprophagy," *Nutrition Reviews* vol. 20, no. 10. New York: The Nutrition Foundation, Inc., 1962.

Bataille, Georges. *Visions of Excess*. Minneapolis: The University of Minnesota Press, 1985.

Bauman, Zygmunt. "The Sweet Scent of Decomposition," *Forget Baudrillard?* (ed. Chris Rojek and Bryan S. Turner). London: Routledge, 1993.

Boies, Lawrence R. *Boies's Fundamentals of Otolaryngology* (5th edition). Philadelphia: W. B. Saunders Company, 1978.

Bose, Girindrashekhar. *Concept of Repression*. Calcutta: G. Bose (printed by Sri Gouranga Press), 1921.

Bosquet, Alain. *Conversations With Dali* (tr. Joachim Neugroschel). New York: E. P. Dutton & Co., Inc., 1969.

Bourke, John G. *Scatalogic Rites of All Nations*. Washington D. C.: W. H. Lowdermilk & Co., 1891. First reprint: New York: Johnson Reprint Corp., 1968.

Brockis, J. Gwynne and Birdwell Finlayson. *Urinary Calculus*. Littleton, Massachusetts: PSG Publishing Company, Inc., 1979.

Brown, Norman O. *Life Against Death*. New York: Vintage Books (Random House), 1959.

Chappell, George S. *Through the Alimentary Canal with a Gun and a Camera*. New York: Frederick A. Stokes Company, 1935.

Chasseguet-Smirgel, Janine. *The Ego Ideal* (tr. Paul Barrows). New York: W. W. Norton & Company, 1984 (original publication: 1975).

Corbin, Alain. *The Foul and the Fragrant*. Cambridge, Massachusetts: Harvard University Press, 1986.

Dali, Salvador. *Diary of a Genius* (tr. Richard Howard). New York: Doubleday & Company, 1965.

Dali, Salvador. *The Secret Life of Salvador Dali* (tr. Haakon M. Chevalier). New York: Dial Press, Burton C. Hoffman, 1942.

Danto, Arthur C. "DeKooning's Three-Seater," *The Nation* vol 240, no. 9. New York: Nation Enterprises, 9 March 1985.

Delaney, Janice. *The Curse*. New York: E. P. Dutton & Co., Inc., 1976.

Dulfano, Mauricio J. *Sputum*. Springfield, Illinois: Charles C. Thomas, Publisher, 1973.

Dundes, Alan. *Life Is Like A Chicken Coop Ladder*. New York: Columbia University Press, 1984.

Ellis, Havelock. *Studies in the Psychology of Sex*. New York: Random House, The Modern Library, Inc., 1936 (orig. pub. 1906).

Ferenczi, Sandor. "The Ontogenesis of the Interest in Money," *Contributions to Psycho-Analysis*. Boston: R. G. Badger, 1916.

Fisher, Carrie. "Madonna: The Rolling Stone Interview," *Rolling Stone* no. 607. New York: Straight Arrow Publishers, Inc., 27 June 1991.

Francia, Luisa. *Dragontime* (tr. Sasha Daucus). Woodstock, New York: Ash Tree Publishing, 1991.

Freud, Sigmund: "Character and Anal Erotism"

(1908), *The Standard Edition of The Complete Psychological Works of Sigmund Freud* (tr. James Strachey). London: The Hogarth Press and the Institute of Psycho-Analysis, 1959.

Freud, Sigmund: "Civilization And Its Discontents" (1930), *The Standard Edition of The Complete Psychological Works of Sigmund Freud* (tr. James Strachey). London: The Hogarth Press and the Institute of Psycho-Analysis, 1959.

Freud, Sigmund. "From the History of an Infantile Neurosis"(1918), *The Standard Edition of The Complete Psychological Works of Sigmund Freud* (tr. James Strachey). London: The Hogarth Press and the Institute of Psycho-Analysis, 1959.

Fromm, Erich. *The Heart of Man*. New York: Harper & Row, Publishers, Inc., 1964.

Fry, Gary F. "Analysis of Prehistoric Coprolites from Utah," *University of Utah Anthropological Papers*, No. 97. Salt Lake City: University of Utah Press, 1977.

Gruson, Lindsey. "Is It Art or Just a Toilet Seat? Bidders to Decide on a deKooning," The New York Times vol. 141, no. 48,846. New York: The New York Times Publishing Company, Inc., 15 January 1992.

Gore, Senator Al. *Earth In The Balance*. New York: Houghton Mifflin Company, 1992.

Hafez, E. S. E. *Human Semen and Fertility Regulation in Men*. St. Louis: The C. V. Mosby Company, 1976.

Hafez, E. S. E. *The Human Vagina*. Amsterdam: Elsevier/North-Holland Biomedical Press, 1978.

Hafez, E. S. E. *Techniques of Human Andrology*. Amsterdam: Elsevier/North-Holland Biomedical Press, 1977.

Hall, W. W. *Health and Disease*. New York: Hurd and Houghton, 1870.

Harding, Richard. *Survival in Space*. London: Routledge, 1989.

Harington, Sir John. *The Metamorphosis of Ajax* (1596), A Critical Annotated Edition by Elizabeth Story Donno. New York: Columbia University Press, 1962.

Hawks, Richard L. and C. Nora Chiang. *Urine Testing for Drugs of Abuse* (NIDA Research Monograph 73). Rockville, Maryland: National Institute on Drug Abuse, U. S. Department of Health and Human Services, 1986.

Hensel, Otto and Richard Weil. *The Urine and Feces in Diagnosis*. Philadelphia: Lea Brothers & Co., 1905.

Horwitz, Tony. "Endangered Feces: Paleo-Scatologist Plumbs Old Privies," *The Wall Street Journal*, Vol. 125, No. 49. New York: Dow Jones & Company, Inc., 9 September 1991.

Ianonne, Paul. "What Every Teenager Should Know About Intercourse During Periods," *Ben Is Dead*, no. 23. Hollywood, California: Ben Is Dead Magazine, 1994.

John Boswell Associates and Sean Kelly. *The Bean Report*. New York: Warner Books, Inc., 1984.

Jung, Carl G. *Memories, Dreams, Reflections* (ed. Aniela Jaffé, tr. Richard and Clara Winston). New York: Vintage Books, A Division of Random House, 1965.

Kellogg, John H. *Colon Hygiene*. Battle Creek, Michigan: Good Health Publishing, 1917.

Khomeini, Ruhollah. *Worship and Self-Development According to the Tahrir al-Wasilah of Ayatullah 'Uzma Imam Khomeini* (tr. Laleh Bakhtiar). Teheran: Foreign Department of Bonyad Ba'that, 1986.

Kimball, Michael. "On Farting," *CoEvolution Quarterly* No. 34. Sausalito, California: POINT, a California nonprofit corporation, 1982.

Kira, Alexander. *The Bathroom: Criteria for Design* (2nd edition). New York: The Viking Press, 1976.

Kubie, Lawrence. "The Fantasy of Dirt," *The Psychoanalytic Quarterly*, Vol. 6. Albany, New York: The Psychoanalytic Quarterly, Inc., 1937.

Kundera, Milan. *The Unbearable Lightness of Being* (tr. Michael Henry Heim). New York: Harper & Row, Publishers, Inc., 1984.

Laden, Karl and Carl B. Felger. *Antiperspirants and Deodorants*. New York: Marcel Dekker, Inc., 1988.

Lavelle, Christopher L. B. *Applied Physiology of the Mouth*. Bristol, England: John Wright and Sons Limited, 1975.

Nohain, Jean and F. Caradec. *Le Petomane 1857-*

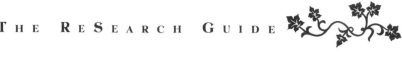
1945 (tr. Warren Tute). London: Souvenir Press Ltd., 1967.

Mack, Alison. *Toilet Learning*. Boston: Little, Brown and Company, 1978.

Mann, Thaddeus and Cecilia Lutwak-Mann. *Male Reproductive Function and Semen*. Berlin: Springer-Verlag, 1981.

Martin, Judith. *Miss Manners' Guide to Excruciatingly Correct Behavior*. New York: Warner Books, Inc., 1983.

Meyer, Kathleen. *How to Shit in the Woods*. Berkeley, California: Ten Speed Press, 1989.

Milder, Benjamin. *The Lacrimal System*. Norwalk, Connecticut: Appleton-Century-Crofts, A Publishing Division of Prentice-Hall, Inc., 1983.

Mithal, C. P. *Urine Therapy*. New Delhi: Pankaj Publications, 1978.

Montaigne, Michel de. *The Complete Essays of Montaigne* (tr. Donald M. Frame). Stanford, California: Stanford University Press, 1958.

Muir, Frank. *An Irreverent and Almost Complete Social History of the Bathroom*. Briarcliff Manor, New York: Stein and Day, 1982.

Mundy, A. R., T. P. Stephenson, and A. J. Wein. *Urodynamics, Principles Practices and Application*. Edinburgh: Churchill Livingstone, 1984.

Neville, Margaret C. and Marianne R. Neifert. *Lactation: Physiology, Nutrition, and Breast-Feeding*. New York: Plenum Press, 1983.

Olds, Sally Wendkos and Marvin S. Eiger. *The Complete Book of Breastfeeding*. New York: Workman Publishing Company, Inc.

Pagel, Walter. *Paracelsus*. Basel, Switzerland: S. Karger AG, 1958.

Parinaud, André. *The Unspeakable Confessions of Salvador Dali* (tr. Harold J. Salemson). New York: William Morrow and Company, Inc., 1976.

Pirsig, Robert. *Zen and the Art of Motorcycle Maintenance*. New York: William Morrow and Company, Inc., 1974.

Profet, Margie. "Menstruation as a Defense Against Pathogens Transported by Sperm," *The Quarterly Review of Biology* vol. 63, no. 3. Chicago: The University of Chicago Press, September 1993.

Reyburn, Wallace. *Flushed With Pride: The Story of Thomas Crapper*. Englewood Cliffs, New Jersey: Prentice-Hall, Inc., 1969.

Reynolds, Reginald. *Cleanliness and Godliness*. London: George Allen & Unwin Ltd., 1943.

Rook, Arthur, D. S. Wilkinson, F. J. G. Ebling, R. H. Champion, and J. L. Burton. *Textbook of Dermatology* (fourth edition). Oxford: Blackwell Scientific Publications, 1986.

Rosebury, Theodor. *Life On Man*. New York: The Viking Press, Inc., 1969.

Rosenthal, Jack, editor. "A Modest Proposal" (editorial), *The New York Times* vol. 140, no. 48,410. New York: The New York Times Publishing Company, Inc., 5 Nov. 1990.

Ross, Doris L. and Ann E. Neely. *Textbook of Urinalysis and Body Fluids*. Norwalk, Connecticut: Appleton-Century-Crofts, 1983.

Ross, W. Donald, Michael Hirt, and Richard Kurtz. "The Fantasy of Dirt and Attitudes Toward Body Products," *The Journal of Nervous and Mental Disease* vol. 146, no. 4. Baltimore: The Williams & Wilkins Co., 1968.

Ross, Harold. "Notes and Comment," *The New Yorker* vol. 10, no. 24. New York: The New Yorker Magazine, Inc., 28 July 1934.

Rozin, Paul and April Fallon. "A Perspective on Disgust," *Psychological Review* vol. 94, no. 1. Washington, D.C.: American Psychological Association, Inc., 1987.

Rozin, Paul, Linda Millman, and Carol Nemeroff. "Operation of the Laws of Sympathetic Magic in Disgust and Other Domains," *Journal of Personality and Social Psychology* vol. 50, no. 4. Washington, D.C.: American Psychological Association, Inc., 1986.

Rozin, Paul, April Fallon, and Mary Lynn Augustoni-Ziskind: "The Child's Conception of Food: The Development of Contamination Sensitivity to 'Disgusting' Substances," *Developmental Psychology* vol. 21. Washington, D.C.: American Psychological Association, Inc., 1985.

Rozin, Paul, April Fallon, and Robin Mondell. "Family Resemblance in Attitudes to Foods," *Developmental Psychology* vol. 20, no. 2. Washington, D.C.: American Psychological Association, Inc., 1984.

Rubin, William S. *Dada, Surrealism, and their Heritage*. New York: The Museum of Modern Art, 1968.

Sabbath, Dan and Mandel Hall. *End Product: The First Taboo*. New York: Urizen Books, 1977.

Salisbury, Harrison E. *The New Emperors*. Boston: Little, Brown and Company, 1992.

Samitz, M. H. *Cutaneous Disorders of the Lower Extremities* (second edition). Philadelphia: J. B. Lippincott Company, 1981.

Sampson, John A. "Peritoneal Endometriosis Due To The Menstrual Dissemination Of Endometrial Tissue Into the Peritoneal Cavity," *The American Journal of Obstetrics and Gynecology* vol. 14, no. 4. St. Louis: The C. V. Mosby Company, October 1927.

Schoenfeld, Eugene. *Dear Doctor Hip Pocrates*. New York: Grove Press, Inc., 1968.

Schultes, Richard E. *Hallucinogenic Plants* (A Golden Guide®). New York: Golden Press, 1976.

Shrager, Sidney. *Scatology in Modern Drama*. New York: Irvington Publishers, Inc., 1982.

Sullivan, David A. (editor). *Lacrimal Glands, Tear Film, and Dry Eye Syndromes: Basic Science and Clinical Relevance*. New York: Plenum Press, 1994.

Twain, Mark. *"1601" and Sketches Old and New*. New York: The Golden Hind Press, 1933.

Vercellini, Paolo, Guido Ragni, Laura Trespidi, Sabina Oldani and Pier Giorgio Crosingani. "Does Contraception Modify the Risk of Endometriosis?," *Human Reproduction* vol 8, no.4. Oxford: Oxford University Press, April 1993.

Walker, Stanley. *Mrs. Astor's Horse*. New York: Frederick A. Stokes Company, 1935.

Waters, Harry F. "Song to an Unsung Hero" (review of Flushed With Pride), *Newsweek* vol. 74, no. 22. Dayton, Ohio: Newsweek, Inc., 1 December 1969.

Weiss, Rick. "Travel Can Be Sickening; Now Scientists Know Why," *The New York Times* vol. 141, no. 48,950. New York: The New York Times Publishing Company, Inc., 28 Apr. 1992.

Wright, Lawrence. *Clean and Decent*. London: Routledge & Kegan Paul Limited, 1960.

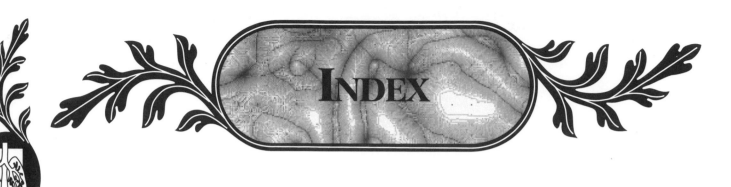

INDEX

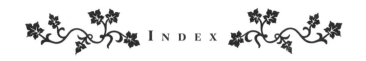
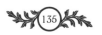

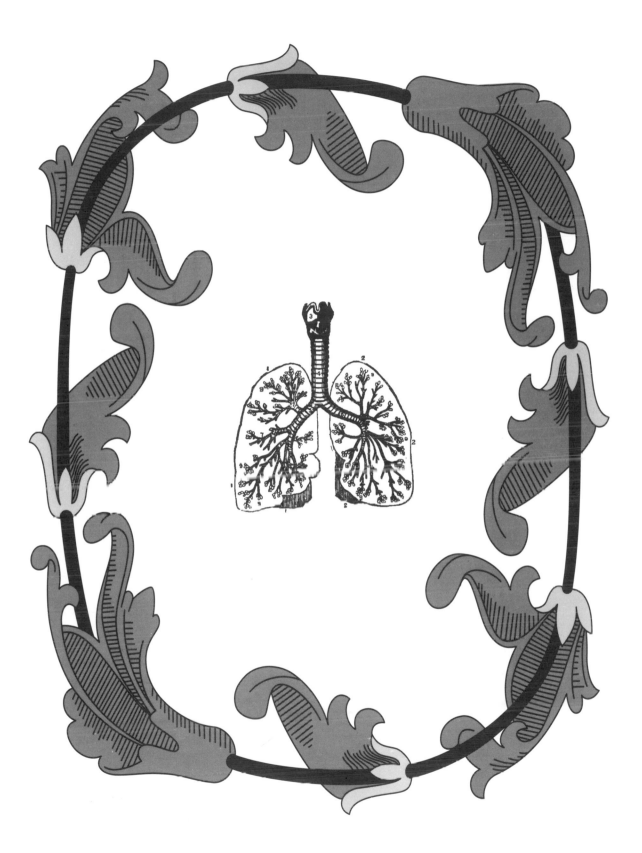

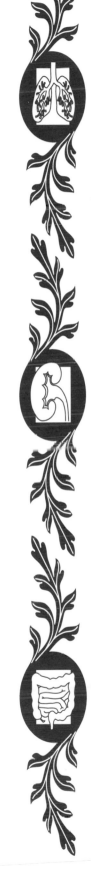

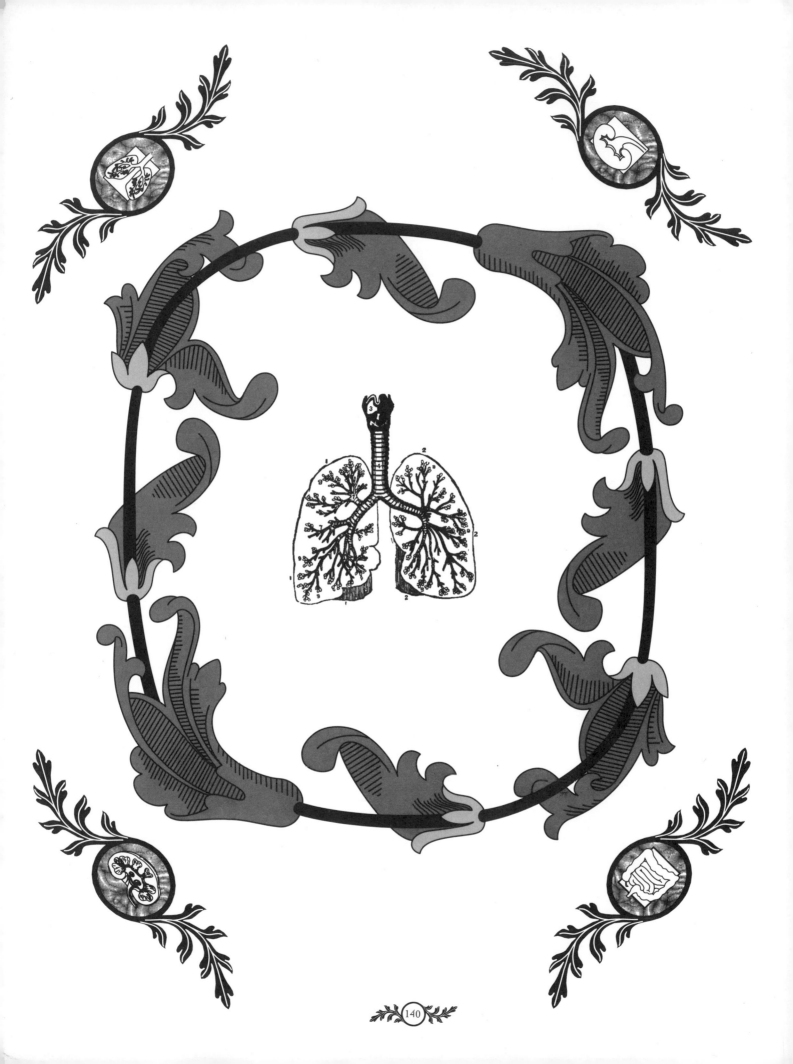